Swallowing – Physiology, Disorders, Diagnosis and Therapy

Gauri Mankekar
Editor

Swallowing – Physiology, Disorders, Diagnosis and Therapy

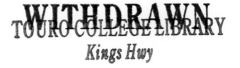
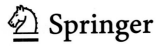 Springer

Editor
Gauri Mankekar
ENT
PD Hinduja Hospital
Mumbai
Maharashtra
India

ISBN 978-81-322-2418-1   ISBN 978-81-322-2419-8   (eBook)
DOI 10.1007/978-81-322-2419-8

Library of Congress Control Number: 2015941276

Springer New Delhi Heidelberg New York Dordrecht London

Printed on acid-free paper

Springer International Publishing AG Switzerland is part of Springer Science+Business Media (www.springer.com)

Foreword

I am a practicing pediatric otolaryngologist at UTMB Health, Galveston, for the past several years. When Dr. Mankekar approached me to write a foreword for her book, I was humbled and felt privileged at the same time. I have known Dr. Mankekar, the editor of this book, for several years now. I was fortunate to work and train under her as a resident otolaryngologist during my early years. She is an excellent physician and surgeon, and undoubtedly she has been the driving force behind the concept and evolution of writing this book. Knowing her I am happy to say that this book will be thorough and clinically relevant.

Swallowing disorders are more common in adults than children. However, a subset of the pediatric population particularly children with reflux, congenital abnormalities such as tracheoesophageal fistula, or children with chemical burn injury to the esophagus tend to have significant swallowing issues. The swallowing mechanism is a highly complex and neurologically regulated process such that varied diseases and conditions can affect swallowing. This book is a comprehensive review of the various swallowing disorders, their diagnosis, and treatment. I really appreciate the fact that there is a separate chapter on neurogenic dysphagia which is a common but difficult to treat problem.

Despite diagnostic and technical advancements, swallowing problems continue to affect a large number of the adults as well as the geriatric population. Many a times consistent collaboration and team work is required amongst the medical doctors, speech and occupational therapists, neurologists, and the surgical team. With the advent of noninvasive techniques to treat dysphagia such as Botox injections and various guidelines outlined by the American Speech Language and Hearing Association (ASHA), this book is timely to give the reader not only an overview of the common causes of dysphagia but also provide up-to-date and current information about the latest modalities of diagnosis and management.

The authors of the various book chapters are renowned physicians and have had a lot of experience in treating swallowing problems. It is a testament to their effort and not at all surprising that this book is well-written, easy to read, and has several treatment algorithms that the reader will definitely benefit from. I am positive that both the beginner and the experienced physician will learn something new that will positively affect their care of such patients.

I hope you enjoy reading the book as much as the authors enjoyed and worked hard to get this information to the readers. Good luck to all the authors and I hope that it serves the readers well.

Galveston, TX, USA   Shraddha Mukerji, MD

Foreword

Dysphagia is a common ENT problem. A multidisciplinary approach has improved care of patients with swallowing disorders, wherein numerous healthcare professionals are involved in its management. A team including otolaryngologists, gastroenterologists, neurologists, radiologists, swallowing therapists, and dietitians is involved in the care of patients with dysphagia. Dr. Gauri Mankekar is a well-known ENT surgeon from Mumbai and has brought together a multidisciplinary team of authors to write on swallowing. The book *Swallowing – Physiology, Disorders, Diagnosis and Therapy* will really help consultant otolaryngologists and PG students in their endeavor to treat swallowing disorders. This book provides a detailed and up-to-date knowledge of the diagnosis and management of dysphagia, with special reference to pediatric dysphagia. I am certain that clinicians will find this a useful clinical reference and utilize it in their day-to-day practice.

Ujjain, MP, India   Sudhakar Vaidya

Preface

Swallowing like breathing is an integral part of our lives. We realize the importance of these functions only when we encounter problems. Although swallowing disorders can affect all age groups, the incidence is higher amongst children and the elderly. Our knowledge about the mechanism of swallowing and related disorders has improved over the past several decades. Advances in endoscopic techniques, manometry, endoscopic ultrasound, and imaging techniques have enabled us to diagnose as well as manage swallowing disorders. Of course, this means that the approach has to be multidisciplinary. The otolaryngologist is often the first to be approached by a patient with a swallowing disorder, but a gastroenterologist may be required to identify and manage the patient with esophageal disorders. Since swallowing involves neuromuscular coordination, a neurologist has to step in and identify the type and level of lesion causing the swallowing disorder, while the radiologist can help identify and document the lesions. An intensivist revives a patient in the intensive care but, on extubating the patient, finds that the patient has dysphagia. Once the problem is identified, the swallowing therapist begins with the rehabilitation and management of the swallowing disorder.

This book provides an overview of swallowing disorders from the perspective of this multidisciplinary team. It is by no means comprehensive. It includes chapters on pediatric dysphagia and dysphagia in the elderly as well as clinical vignettes which may help pediatricians, internists, neurologists, gastroenterologists, and swallowing therapists in their practice.

Mumbai, India   Gauri Mankekar

Acknowledgments

Editing a book with contributions from busy clinicians all over the world is a herculean task. But I had tremendous support and would like to acknowledge all those involved.

Firstly, the contributors, Dr. Kashmira Chavan, Dr. Rajesh Sainani, Dr. Charu Sankhla, Dr. Devaki Dewan, Dr. Simran Singh, Ms Justine Joan Sheppard, Ms Georgia Malandraki, Ms Dalia Noguiera, and Ms Rita Patel for writing the chapters related to their specialties. All of them have very busy schedules but somehow found the time to contribute, and I thank them.

Mrs. Dalvi, retired lecturer, Speech Language Pathology, Ali Yavar Jung National Institute for the Hearing Handicapped, Mumbai, India, was the first person who aroused my curiosity about the management of swallowing disorders. A dedicated therapist, she helped rehabilitate several patients with dysphagias.

My patients, my husband Dinesh Vartak, and my mom who have been a constant source of inspiration.

And last but not the least, the most important contributors to this venture – the team at Springer, India, who have made this book a reality – thank you.

Contents

Anatomy of Swallowing

1

Kashmira Chavan

Introduction

The complex function of swallowing involves anatomical structures extending from the oral cavity (lips, teeth, tongue, cheeks, oral vestibular, palate and palatal arches) to the pharynx, larynx, hypopharynx and the esophagus.

The Oral Cavity (Fig. 1.1)

The oral cavity is the initial site for the processing of food. It extends from the lips to the pharynx. The oral cavity is divided by the dental arches (formed by the teeth and alveoli) into two parts:

1. Outer vestibule
2. Inner oral cavity proper

The Oral Vestibule [1, 2]

The part of the oral cavity lying between the dental arches and the deep surfaces of the cheeks and lips is referred to as the oral vestibule. It is lined by mucous membrane. The parotid duct and the labial, buccal, and molar glands open into the oral vestibule. Anteriorly, it communicates exteriorly via the oral fissure and posteriorly with the oral cavity proper.

K. Chavan, MBBS, DNB
ENT, Dr. L.H. Hiranandani Hospital, Powai, Mumbai, India
e-mail: kashuc@yahoo.com

© Springer India 2015
G. Mankekar (ed.), *Swallowing – Physiology, Disorders, Diagnosis and Therapy*,
DOI 10.1007/978-81-322-2419-8_1

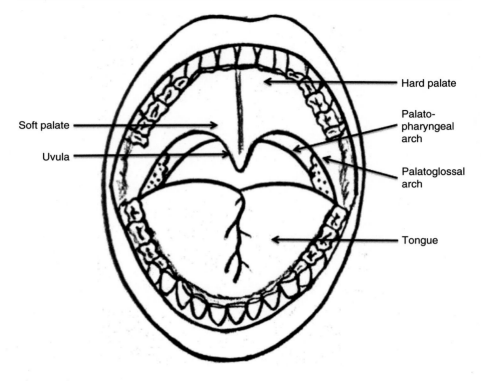

Soft palate

Uvula

Hard palate

Palato-
pharyngeal
arch

Palatoglossal
arch

Tongue

Fig. 1.1 The oral cavity

The Lips

The lips surround the oral fissure and are composed of the orbicularis oris muscle
and submucosa (containing mucous labial glands, labial vessels, nerves, fatty
tissues). They are lined externally by skin and internally by mucous membrane.
Contraction of the orbicularis oris narrows the mouth and closes the lips like a
sphincter, thus retaining the food bolus in the mouth [1, 2].

Oral Cavity Proper [2]

Boundaries
Roof: The hard and soft palates separate the oral cavity from the nasal cavities.
Floor: The floor is formed by the tongue and a muscular diaphragm formed by the
    muscles in the floor of the oral cavity.
Lateral walls: The lateral walls are formed by the cheeks.
Posteriorly: It opens into the pharynx at the oropharyngeal isthmus, which is bound
    superiorly by the soft palate, inferiorly by the tongue, and laterally on either
    sides by the faucial pillars formed by the palatoglossal (anterior arch) and
    palatopharyngeal (posterior arch) muscles.
Anteriorly: It communicates with the oral vestibule.

Cheeks

The cheeks form the lateral walls of the oral cavity and are continuous with the lips at the nasolabial sulcus. Each cheek is composed of skin, superficial fascia, parotid duct, mucous buccal and molar glands, vessels, nerves, lymphatics, fat, submucosa, and mucosa. The muscle of the cheek, the buccinator, arises from the pterygomandibular raphe and the posterior part of the maxilla and mandible opposite the molar teeth. The fibers of the buccinator together with fibers from the orbicularis oris insert into the lips [2]. The parotid duct pierces the buccinator muscle before opening into the oral cavity opposite the second upper molar tooth. This buccinator derives its nerve supply from the facial nerve. During mastication, the buccinators contract, press the cheeks against the teeth, and make the cheeks taut, thus preventing accumulation of food between the teeth and the cheeks [1–3].

Hard Palate [2]

The hard palate forms the partition between the oral and nasal cavities and is composed of the palatine processes of each maxilla anteriorly and the horizontal plates of each palatine bone posteriorly. Its posterior margin gives attachment to the soft palate. The alveolar arch lies anterior and lateral to the oral surface of the hard palate.

Soft Palate

The soft palate separates the nasopharynx from the oropharynx. It is lined by mucous membrane and consists of palatine aponeurosis (flattened tensor veli palatini tendon), taste buds, mucous glands, and muscles. The palatine aponeurosis splits in the midline to enclose the musculus uvulae, which forms the posterior free hanging midline projection, the uvula [1].

The various muscles involved with the mobility of the soft palate are listed in Table 1.1 [2].

The soft palate on elevation comes into contact with Passavant's ridge, closing the pharyngeal isthmus during swallowing. This separates the nasopharynx from the oropharynx, thus preventing nasal regurgitation. Depression of the soft palate closes the oropharyngeal isthmus.

Tongue

The tongue is a muscular structure forming the floor of the oral cavity. In addition to being an organ of taste, it plays an important role in the oral phase of swallowing. A median connective tissue septum divides the tongue into right and left halves, each half containing paired intrinsic and extrinsic muscles [1, 2]. Figure 1.2 shows some of the various tongue muscles.

Table 1.1 Muscles of the soft palate [2]

Muscle	Origin	Insertion	Innervation	Function
Tensor veli palatini	(A) Fibrous part of pharyngotympanic tube (B) Scaphoid fossa of sphenoid bone (C) Spine of sphenoid	Palatine aponeurosis	Mandibular nerve [V3] via the branch to the medial pterygoid muscle	(A) Tenses the soft palate (B) Opens the pharyngotympanic tube for pressure equalization
Levator veli palatini *Lies deep to the tensor palatini*	Petrous part of the temporal bone anterior to opening for the carotid canal	Superior surface of the palatine aponeurosis	Vagus nerve [X] via the pharyngeal branch to the pharyngeal plexus	Only muscle to elevate the soft palate above the neutral position
Palatopharyngeus *A few fibers of the palatopharyngeus along with some fibers of the superior constrictor muscle form a ring around the posterior and lateral walls of the nasopharyngeal isthmus. On soft palate elevation, this muscle band forms a ridge called Passavant's ridge*	Superior surface of the palatine aponeurosis	Pharyngeal wall	Vagus nerve [X] via the pharyngeal branch to the pharyngeal plexus	(A) Depresses the soft palate (B) Moves the palatopharyngeal arch toward midline (C) Elevates the pharynx
Palatoglossus	Inferior surface of the palatine aponeurosis	Lateral margin of the tongue	Vagus nerve [X] via the pharyngeal branch to the pharyngeal plexus	(A) Depresses the palate (B) Moves the palatoglossal arch toward midline (C) Elevates back of the tongue
Musculus uvulae	Posterior nasal spine of the hard palate	Connective tissue of the uvula	Vagus nerve [X] via the pharyngeal branch to the pharyngeal plexus	(A) Elevates and retracts the uvula (B) Thickens the central region of the soft palate

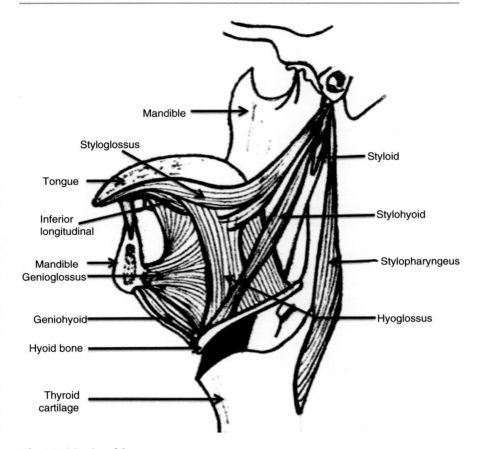

Fig. 1.2 Muscles of the tongue

Intrinsic muscles (originate and insert within the tongue):

- Superior longitudinal
- Inferior longitudinal
- Transverse
- Vertical

Extrinsic muscles (originate outside the tongue and insert within the substance of the tongue):

- Genioglossus
- Hyoglossus
- Styloglossus
- Palatoglossus

The base of the tongue is attached to the epiglottis by the median and lateral glossoepiglottic folds. The vallecula lies between the median and lateral glossoepiglottic folds on either side. The tongue is attached to the mandible by the genioglossus, to the hyoid bone by the hyoglossus, to the styloid process by the styloglossus, and to the palate by the palatoglossus. The extrinsic muscles protrude, retract, depress, and elevate the tongue, while the intrinsic muscles alter the shape of the tongue by lengthening, shortening, curling, and uncurling its apex and sides and flattening and rounding its surface [1, 2]. They thus help in performing finer movements of the tongue during speech, mastication, and swallowing.

Innervation of the Tongue

All the tongue muscles are innervated by the hypoglossal nerve, except the palatoglossus which is innervated by the vagus nerve via its pharyngeal branch to the pharyngeal plexus [1, 2]. Sensory fibers from the anterior portion of the tongue are carried by the lingual nerve, a branch of the trigeminal nerve. Special sensory taste fibers from the anterior two-thirds of the tongue leave the tongue and travel along with the lingual nerve before traveling via the chorda tympani nerve, a branch of the facial nerve. Special sensory taste fibers from the posterior one-third of the tongue are supplied by the glossopharyngeal nerve.

Muscles of Mastication

The muscles of mastication are responsible for the movements of the mandible during swallowing and speech. The various muscles are listed in Table 1.2 [2].

Unilateral contraction of the pterygoid muscles leads to contralateral movement of the mandible. Coordinated movements on both sides result in proper chewing of the food bolus [2].

Teeth and Dentition [1, 2]

The teeth play an important role in mastication. The teeth are embedded in a horseshoe-shaped bony ridge called alveolar process in the maxilla and mandible. Loss of teeth results in resorption of the alveolar bone and disappearance of the alveolar arches. The teeth and adjacent alveolar regions are surrounded by the gingivae (gums). Two sets of teeth develop in humans, deciduous teeth and permanent teeth. The deciduous teeth erupt from the gingivae between 6 months and 2 years of age [1]. Premolars and third molars are absent in children. The 20 deciduous teeth consist of two incisors, one canine, and two molar teeth in each half of the upper and lower jaws. These are replaced by the permanent incisor, canine, and premolar teeth. The jaws elongate forward to accommodate the permanent molar teeth, which erupt posterior to the deciduous molars [1, 2]. Replacement of the deciduous teeth by permanent teeth begins at about 6 years of age and continues into adulthood [2].

Table 1.2 Muscles of mastication [2]

Muscle	Origin	Insertion	Innervation	Function
Masseter	Superficial layer: maxillary process of the zygomatic bone, anterior two-thirds of the zygomatic process of the maxilla. Deep layer: medial aspect of the zygomatic arch and the posterior part of its inferior margin	Superficial fibers: angle of the mandible and lower part of the ramus of the mandible. Deep fibers: central and upper parts of the ramus of the mandible and the coronoid process	Masseteric nerve from the anterior trunk of the mandibular nerve [V3]	Elevation of the mandible
Temporalis	Bony surface of the temporal fossa superior to the inferior temporal line, attached laterally to the deep surface of the temporalis fascia	Fibers converge inferiorly to form a tendon passing between the zygomatic arch and the infratemporal crest of the greater wing of the sphenoid to insert into margins and deep surface of the coronoid process and the anterior border of the ramus of the mandible	Deep temporal nerves from the anterior trunk of the mandibular nerve [V3]	Elevation and retraction of the mandible; side-to-side movements of the mandible
Lateral pterygoid	Upper head: roof of the infratemporal fossa. Lower head: lateral surface of the lateral pterygoid plate	Pterygoid fovea of the neck of the mandible; capsule of the temporomandibular joint near the internal attachment of the capsule to the articular disk	Nerve to the lateral pterygoid from the anterior trunk of the mandibular nerve [V3]	Protrusion and side-to-side movements of the mandible; pulls the articular disk and head of the mandible forward onto the articular tubercle
Medial pterygoid	Superficial head: tuberosity and pyramidal process of the maxilla. Deep head: medial surface of the lateral pterygoid plate; pyramidal process of the palatine bone	Medial surface of angle and the ramus of the mandible	Nerve to the medial pterygoid from the mandibular nerve [V3]	Elevation and side-to-side movements of the mandible; assists the lateral pterygoid in mandibular protrusion

A fully dentured adult jaw consists of 32 teeth. There are 16 teeth each in the upper and lower jaw – the central incisor, the lateral incisor, the canine, the first premolar, the second premolar, the first molar, the second molar, and the third molar.

The shape of each tooth determines its function. The incisors (front teeth) have one root and a chisel-shaped crown, which can "cut." The canines have a crown with a single pointed cusp with which they can grasp. The premolars have a crown with two cusps, while the crowns of molars have three–five cusps for grinding [2]. Irregular dentition, loss of teeth, or diseases of the gums and teeth can interfere with the process of mastication and bolus formation.

Salivary Glands

The minor and the major salivary glands secrete saliva into the oral cavity. The minor salivary glands situated in the submucosa or mucosa of the oral epithelium lining the tongue, palate, cheeks, and lips open into the oral cavity directly or via small ducts. The major salivary glands are the parotid, the submandibular, and the sublingual salivary glands.

Parotid Gland

The parotid gland is located between the ramus of the mandible anteriorly, the sternocleidomastoid muscle posteriorly, and the external auditory meatus and the root of the zygoma superiorly. It overlies the masseter muscle anteriorly and the posterior belly of the digastric muscle posteriorly.

The parotid gland encloses the external carotid artery and the retromandibular vein. The extracranial facial nerve passes in between the superficial and deep lobes of the parotid gland. The parotid duct (Stenson's duct) passes anteriorly over the external surface of the masseter muscle, turns medially to penetrate the buccinator muscle, and opens into the oral cavity opposite to the crown of the second upper molar tooth.

Submandibular Gland

The submandibular gland is situated within the submandibular triangle. The superficial part of the gland lies in the submandibular fossa on the medial surface of the mandible, while the deeper portion loops around the mylohyoid muscle to lie within the floor of the oral cavity.

The submandibular duct (Wharton's duct) arises from the deeper portion of the gland and opens lateral to frenulum of the tongue in the anterior portion of the floor of the oral cavity, behind the incisors.

Sublingual Gland

The sublingual salivary gland is situated lateral to the submandibular duct in the floor of the mouth. The sublingual glands drain into the floor of the oral cavity via numerous small sublingual ducts which open onto the sublingual fold.

Larynx

The larynx is composed of a cartilaginous framework held together by muscles and ligaments. The laryngeal cavity lies in continuity with the pharynx superiorly and the trachea inferiorly.

Laryngeal Cartilages [1, 2]

- *Unpaired cartilages:* thyroid, cricoid, and epiglottis
- *Paired cartilages:* arytenoid, corniculate, and cuneiform

Ligaments [1, 2]

- *Extrinsic ligaments:* thyrohyoid ligament, hyoepiglottic ligament, and cricotracheal ligament
- *Intrinsic ligament:* fibroelastic membrane of the larynx which is composed of two parts:
  - Cricothyroid ligament: Attached anteriorly to the thyroid cartilage and posteriorly to the vocal processes of the arytenoid cartilages. The free margin between these two attachments forms the vocal ligament, which constitutes the true vocal cords.
  - Quadrangular membrane: Its lower free margin forms the vestibular ligament, which constitutes the false vocal cords.

Laryngeal Muscles

Intrinsic Muscles [1, 2]
These are the muscles whose origin and insertion are both within the laryngeal framework:

- Cricothyroid
- Posterior cricoarytenoid
- Lateral cricoarytenoid

- Transverse arytenoid
- Oblique arytenoid
- Aryepiglotticus
- Thyroarytenoid
- Vocalis

Function
The intrinsic laryngeal muscles are responsible for tensing and relaxing the vocal ligaments, opening and closing the rima glottidis, adjusting the laryngeal vestibule dimensions, and facilitating closure of the rima vestibuli and laryngeal inlet.

Extrinsic Muscles [1, 2]
The extrinsic muscles are those which have an attachment to a site within the larynx and another outside the larynx (e.g., hyoid bone). They are divided into:

- *Suprahyoid muscles* (superior to the hyoid bone):
  - Stylohyoid
  - Mylohyoid
  - Geniohyoid
  - Digastric

Function
The suprahyoid muscles elevate the hyoid bone and the larynx.

- *Infrahyoid muscles* (inferior to the hyoid bone):
  - Sternothyroid
  - Sternohyoid
  - Thyrohyoid
  - Omohyoid

Function
The infrahyoid muscles depress the larynx and the hyoid bone.

Laryngeal Adductor Reflex

The laryngeal adductor reflex (LAR) [4], also called the glottic closure reflex, is a brainstem-mediated, involuntary reflex arc, which prevents substances from inappropriately entering the airway. The LAR is a bilateral thyroarytenoid (TA) muscle response to mechanical or chemical irritation of the laryngeal mucosa. The afferent limb of this reflex arc is formed by the superior laryngeal nerve, while the recurrent laryngeal nerve acts as the efferent limb [4].

The knowledge about LAR continues to evolve with some studies reporting that the response of the TA muscle to air pressure (air puff stimuli) is physiologically different from the laryngeal adductor reflex that occurs in response to electrical stimulation of the superior laryngeal nerve [5]. During speech and swallowing, mechanoreceptors in the laryngeal mucosa are subjected to pressures generated by vocal fold closure, which are similar to these air puff stimuli [5].

During swallowing, the action of the intrinsic and extrinsic muscles results in the closure of the rima glottides and the rima vestibule. Narrowing of the laryngeal inlet occurs along with upward and forward movement of the larynx. As a result the epiglottis moves toward the arytenoid cartilages with narrowing down or closure of the laryngeal inlet. Elevation of the larynx by the suprahyoid muscles also opens the pharyngoesophageal segment. This sequence of events directs the solids and liquids through the piriform fossae into the esophagus and prevents them from entering the airway [1–3]. Figure 1.3 shows the relations of the oral cavity, larynx, pharynx, and esophagus.

Pharynx [1, 2]

The pharynx is a musculofascial half-cylinder attached above to the skull base and is continuous below with the esophagus, at the level of C6 vertebra. The pharyngeal cavity is a common pathway for air and food.

Anteriorly the pharyngeal walls are attached to the margins of the nasal cavities, oral cavity, and larynx, which communicate with the pharynx. Based on their relation, the pharynx is subdivided into three regions, the nasopharynx, oropharynx, and laryngopharynx (hypopharynx) (Fig. 1.3).

Nasopharynx

The nasopharynx is the superior most part of the pharynx. Its roof slopes downward and is formed cranially to caudally by the basisphenoid, the basiocciput, and the anterior aspect of the first two cervical vertebrae. The hard palate and Passavant's muscle form the level of its inferior margin. It is continuous below with the oropharynx and communicates anteriorly with the nasal cavities. The lateral walls are formed by the margins of the superior constrictor muscle and the pharyngobasilar fascia. The pharyngeal tonsils lie in the mucosa in the midline of the roof of the nasopharynx. The Eustachian tube openings lie in the posterolateral walls of the nasopharynx on either side. The Eustachian tube opening along with the cartilaginous Eustachian tube, the levator veli palatini muscle, and the overlying mucosa forms the torus tubarius. A recess, the fossa of Rosenmüller, is situated slightly posterior and superior to the torus tubarius. Mucosal folds in the nasopharynx cover the salpingopharyngeus (salpingopharyngeal fold) and levator veli palatini muscles.

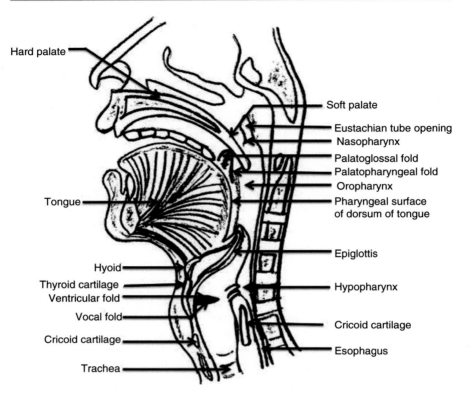

Hard palate

Soft palate

Eustachian tube opening
Nasopharynx

Palatoglossal fold
Palatopharyngeal fold
Oropharynx

Tongue

Pharyngeal surface
of dorsum of tongue

Epiglottis

Hyoid
Thyroid cartilage
Ventricular fold

Hypopharynx

Vocal fold

Cricoid cartilage
Cricoid cartilage

Esophagus

Trachea

Fig. 1.3 Sagittal view showing the relations between the oral cavity, pharynx, larynx, and esophagus

The two muscles open the cartilaginous end of the Eustachian tube by pulling in opposite directions during swallowing. This helps in pressure equalization between the middle ear and the nasopharynx.

Oropharynx

The oropharynx is the region of the pharynx posterior to the oral cavity. It extends from the inferior level of the soft palate to the upper margin of the epiglottis. Its posterior wall is anterior to the second and third cervical vertebrae. It includes the posterior one-third of the tongue (tongue base with collection of lymphoid tissue, the lingual tonsils), palatine tonsils, soft palate, oropharyngeal mucosa, and constrictor muscles. The anterior palatoglossal arch (overlying the palatoglossus muscle) and the posterior palatopharyngeal arch (overlying the palatopharyngeus muscle) are present in the lateral oropharyngeal wall. The palatine tonsils lie in the tonsillar fossa between the two arches (Figs. 1.1 and 1.3).

Hypopharynx

The hypopharynx, or laryngopharynx, extends from the level of the hyoid bone (and valleculae) to the cricopharyngeus. It is continuous superiorly with the oropharynx and inferiorly with the cervical esophagus (level of C6). The posterior oropharyngeal wall continues inferiorly as the posterior wall of the hypopharynx, behind which lies the retropharyngeal space.

The pyriform sinus is a pear-shaped anterolateral recess situated on either side of the hypopharynx. It is related anteriorly to the posterior paraglottic space of the larynx. The apex of the pyriform sinus lies at the level of the true vocal cord. The lateral wall of the pyriform sinus is formed above by the thyrohyoid membrane and below by the thyroid cartilage. The lateral surface of the aryepiglottic fold forms its medial wall. During the process of swallowing, solids and liquids are directed via the pyriform sinuses into the cervical esophagus.

The postcricoid region is the anterior wall of the lower hypopharynx and extends from the level of the cricoarytenoid joints to the lower edge of the cricoid cartilage.

The pharyngeal wall consists of four layers from inside out: mucous membrane, pharyngobasilar fascia, muscular layer, and buccopharyngeal fascia. The muscular layer consists of an outer circular and an inner longitudinal muscle layer.

Circular Muscle Layer

This layer is formed by paired superior, middle, and inferior constrictor muscles (Fig. 1.4). The superior constrictor muscle arises from pterygomandibular raphe, adjacent part of the mandible, and pterygoid hamulus; the middle constrictor arises from the upper margin of the greater horn of hyoid bone and adjacent margins of lesser horn and stylohyoid ligament. The inferior constrictor muscle arises from the cricoid cartilage, oblique line of thyroid cartilage, and a ligament extending between these attachments and crosses the cricothyroid muscle. The inferior constrictor muscle is made up of two parts, the superior thyropharyngeus and the inferior cricopharyngeus. A small triangular area of dehiscence called "Killian's dehiscence" is present between the two parts. The fibers of the cricopharyngeus are continuous with the circular muscle fibers of the esophagus [6]. All the three constrictors insert posteriorly into the median pharyngeal raphe. They overlap each other from below upward.

Innervation of the Constrictor Muscles

The three constrictor muscles are innervated by the pharyngeal branch of the vagus nerve (cranial nerve X).

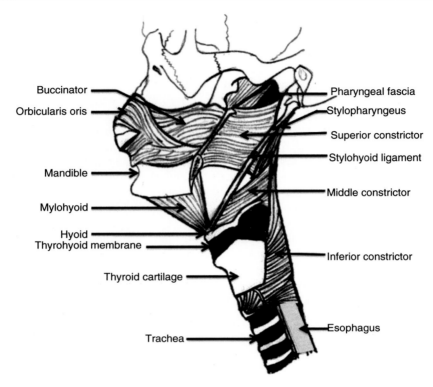

Fig. 1.4 The constrictor muscles of the pharynx (*lateral view*)

Function

Contraction of the muscles leads to constriction of the pharynx. Sequential contraction of the constrictor muscles from above downward results in the propulsion of the food bolus from the pharynx to the esophagus.

Longitudinal Muscle Layer

This layer is formed by the stylopharyngeus (arises from the medial side of base of the styloid process), the salpingopharyngeus (arises from the inferior aspect of the pharyngeal end of the pharyngotympanic tube), and the palatopharyngeus muscles (arises from the upper surface of the palatine aponeurosis) [2]. They insert into the pharyngeal wall.

Innervation

The stylopharyngeus is supplied by the glossopharyngeal nerve, while the salpingopharyngeus and the palatopharyngeus are supplied by the vagus nerve.

Function

The longitudinal muscles elevate the pharyngeal wall or pull the pharyngeal wall up and over a bolus of food passing through the pharynx into the esophagus [2].

Various structures pass through the gaps between the pharyngeal muscles [1, 2]. The pharyngeal wall is deficient between the skull base and the upper margin of the superior constrictor muscle and is completed by the pharyngeal fascia. The tensor and levator veli palatini muscles of the soft palate, the Eustachian tube, and the ascending palatine artery pass through this gap.

The stylopharyngeus muscle and glossopharyngeal nerve pass through the gap between the superior and middle constrictors and the posterior border of the mylohyoid muscle.

The internal laryngeal nerve and superior laryngeal vessels pass through the gap between the middle and inferior constrictors by piercing the thyrohyoid membrane.

The recurrent laryngeal nerve and the inferior laryngeal vessels pass through the gap between the inferior border of the inferior constrictor and the esophagus.

Esophagus [1, 2]

The esophagus is a muscular tube, about 23–25 cm, extending from the pharynx to the stomach. It begins at the inferior border of the cricoid cartilage, opposite C6 vertebra, and ends at the cardiac opening of the stomach, opposite T11 vertebra. It has three constrictions, the first at the cricopharyngeal sphincter (15 cm from the incisors), the second where it is crossed by the aortic arch and the left main bronchus (23 cm from the incisors), and the third where it pierces the diaphragm (40 cm from the incisors) [2].

The esophageal wall is made up of four layers. From outside in, these are as follows:

- Outer fibrous layer
- Muscular layer (outer longitudinal layer and inner circular layer which is continuous with the inferior constrictor muscle of the pharynx)
- Submucous or areolar layer (consists of blood vessels, nerves, mucous glands)
- Internal mucosal layer (covered throughout with a thick layer of stratified squamous epithelium with minute papillae on the surface)

The muscularis mucosae, a layer of longitudinally arranged non-striped muscular fibers, lies between the areolar layer and the mucosal layer. This layer is more prominent in the lower portion of the esophagus.

Upper Esophageal Sphincter

The cricopharyngeus, which originates from the cricoid cartilage, along with the inferior constrictor muscle of the pharynx, and the upper end of the esophagus contribute to the functioning of the upper esophageal sphincter (UES) [7, 8]. The UES is in a state of constant contraction. Coordinated contraction and relaxation of the UES allow the passage of food from the pharynx to the esophagus [7]. The UES derives its nerve supply from the pharyngeal plexus. Innervation of the cricopharyngeus has been a subject of controversy, with some suggesting the recurrent laryngeal nerve as a source of innervation. However recurrent laryngeal paralysis is not associated with UES contractile dysfunction [8]. Some studies have suggested that the cricopharyngeus has double innervation from the recurrent laryngeal and the superior laryngeal nerve, which helps in laryngopharyngeal coordination, especially during swallowing [9].

Lower Esophageal Sphincter [7]

The lower esophageal sphincter is not a well-defined anatomic structure, but a 2–4 cms zone of increased pressure at the lower end of the esophagus. It relaxes during swallowing to allow the food contents to enter the stomach.

Embryology and Development [2, 10]

The anatomy of the swallowing passage differs in infants and adults. In infants, the teeth are not yet erupted, the hard palate is flatter, and the hyoid bone and the larynx are at a higher position in the neck (C2–C3 level). The epiglottis as a result touches the posterior end of the soft palate. The larynx is thus in direct communication with the nasopharynx, but the oropharynx is closed away from the airway during swallowing (Fig. 1.5). This prevents food from entering the airway and protects the infant from aspiration.

During the second year of life, the neck elongates and the larynx starts descending to a lower position. In adults, as a result, the epiglottis is no longer in contact with the soft palate, and the pharynx elongates vertically and becomes a part of the airway. These developmental changes increase the risk of aspiration in adults.

Nerves Involved in Swallowing

Various cranial nerves are responsible for the motor and sensory supply of the swallowing pathway.

Trigeminal Nerve [1, 2]

The trigeminal nerve has both motor and sensory components. The motor fibers, through the mandibular division [V3], innervate the four muscles of mastication (temporalis, masseter, and medial and lateral pterygoids), the tensor tympani, the tensor veli palatini, the anterior belly of the digastric muscle, and the mylohyoid

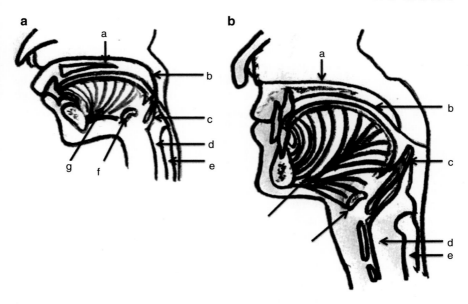

Fig. 1.5 Difference between infant (**a**) and adult (**b**) swallowing passages. Note in (**a**), the palate is flatter, the epiglottis touches the soft palate, and the hyoid is at a higher position. In (**b**), the palate is more curved, the epiglottis and palate are not in contact, and the oral cavity is larger. *a* hard palate, *b* soft palate, *c* epiglottis, *d* larynx, *e* esophagus, *f* hyoid bone, *g* tongue

muscles. The mandibular nerve [V3] also receives sensory branches from the lower lip, the anterior two-thirds of the tongue, the teeth of the lower jaw, and the mucous membranes of the cheek.

Facial Nerve [1, 2]

The motor component of the facial nerve innervates the muscles of the face including the buccinators and orbicularis oris and the stylohyoid and posterior belly of digastric, which elevate the hyoid bone. It carries taste sensations from the anterior two-thirds of the tongue via the chorda tympani. Secretomotor fibers of the facial nerve supply the lacrimal gland and the submandibular and sublingual salivary glands.

Glossopharyngeal Nerve [1, 2]

The glossopharyngeal nerve carries sensory fibers from posterior one-third of the tongue, palatine tonsils, and oropharynx and taste sensations from the posterior one-third of the tongue. The parasympathetic fibers are secretomotor to the parotid gland. It carries motor fibers to the stylopharyngeus muscle. It also contributes to the pharyngeal plexus.

Vagus Nerve [1, 2]

The vagus nerve arises as rootlets from the medulla in the groove between the olive and the inferior peduncle. After exiting the skull base through the jugular foramen, it passes vertically down into the neck, within the carotid sheath, lying between the internal jugular vein and internal carotid artery up to the upper border of the thyroid cartilage. It then descends between the internal jugular vein and the common carotid artery to the root of the neck.

The pharyngeal branch of the vagus passes across the internal carotid artery to the upper border of the middle constrictor muscle of the pharynx, where it communicates with branches from the glossopharyngeal, sympathetic fibers, and the external laryngeal nerve to form the pharyngeal plexus. Branches from this plexus supply the muscles and mucous membrane of the pharynx and the muscles of the soft palate, except the tensor veli palatini.

The superior laryngeal branch of the vagus along with a branch from the superior cervical ganglion of the sympathetic chain descends along the pharynx, behind the internal carotid artery, and divides into two branches, external and internal.

The external laryngeal branch descends on the larynx, beneath the sternothyroid, to supply the cricothyroid muscle. Branches from the external laryngeal nerve contribute to the pharyngeal plexus and supply the inferior constrictor muscle of the pharynx. The internal branch descends to the thyrohyoid membrane and pierces it along with the superior laryngeal artery, to supply the mucous membrane of the larynx. Some branches supply the epiglottis, epiglottic glands, tongue base, and the mucous membrane of the larynx up to the vocal cords. A branch of the internal laryngeal nerve joins the recurrent laryngeal nerve.

The recurrent laryngeal nerve arises, on the right side, in front of the subclavian artery and winds around it, ascending obliquely lateral to the trachea and posterior to the common carotid artery. On the left side, it winds around the aorta and ascends lateral to the trachea. It ascends through the tracheoesophageal grove on both sides, under the inferior constrictor muscle of the pharynx, and enters the larynx behind the cricothyroid joint. It supplies all the muscles of the larynx except the cricothyroid. It communicates with the internal branch of the superior laryngeal nerve and supplies the mucous membrane of the lower portion of the larynx.

As the recurrent laryngeal nerve ascends in the neck, it supplies the mucous membrane and muscular layer of the esophagus (via the esophageal plexus), gives out branches to the tracheal mucous membrane and muscles, and some branches to the inferior constrictor muscle of the pharynx.

Hypoglossal Nerve [1, 2]

The hypoglossal nerve arises as several rootlets from the anterior surface of the medulla, passes across the posterior cranial fossa, and exits the skull base through the hypoglossal canal. It supplies all the intrinsic and most of the extrinsic muscles of the tongue (styloglossus, hyoglossus, and genioglossus). It joins with branches from the second and third cervical nerves, just below the middle of the neck, to form a loop, the ansa cervicalis. Branches from this loop supply the sternohyoid, the sternothyroid, and the inferior belly of the omohyoid.

As in the case of any other system in the body, knowledge of the anatomy of the swallowing pathway would make it easier to understand the actual mechanism of swallowing, which has been discussed in the chapter on the physiology of swallowing.

References

1. Gray H. Oral cavity. In: Standring S, editor. Gray's Anatomy, 40th ed. Edinburgh: Churchill Livingstone. 2008.
2. Drake R, Vogl A, Mitchell A. Gray's anatomy for students. 2nd ed. Philadelphia: Churchill Livingstone; 2009.
3. Merati A, Bielamowicz S, editors. Textbook of laryngology. San Diego: Plural Publishing; 2006.
4. Domer A, Kuhn M, Belafsky P. Neurophysiology and clinical implications of the laryngeal adductor reflex. Curr Otorhinolaryngol Rep. 2013;1:178–82.
5. Bhabu P, Poletto C, Mann E, Bielamowicz S, Ludlow CL. Thyroarytenoid muscle responses to air pressure stimulation of the laryngeal mucosa in humans. Ann Otol Rhinol Laryngol. 2003;112(10):834–40.
6. Gleeson M, Browning GG, Burton MJ, Clarke R, John H, Jones NS, Lund VJ, Luxon LM, Watkinson JC. Scott-Brown's otorhinolaryngology, head and neck surgery. 7th ed. London: Hodder Arnold; 2008.
7. Bailey BJ, Johnson JT, Newlands SD. Head & neck surgery–otolaryngology, vol. 1. Philadelphia: Lippincott Williams and Wilkins; 1993.
8. Shaker R, Belafsky PC, Postma GN. Caryn Easterling principles of deglutition: a multidisciplinary text for swallowing and its disorders. New York: Springer; 2013.
9. Prades JM, et al. The cricopharyngeal muscle and the laryngeal nerves: contribution to the functional anatomy of swallowing. Morphologie. 2009;93(301):35–41.
10. Palmer JB, Matsuo K. Anatomy and physiology of feeding and swallowing: normal and abnormal. Phys Med Rehabil Clin N Am. 2008;19:691–707.

Physiology of Swallowing and Esophageal Function Tests

2

Gauri Mankekar and Kashmira Chavan

Introduction

Swallowing is the continuous process of deglutition from placement of the food in the mouth, its manipulation in the oral cavity, and its passage through the oral cavity, pharynx, and esophagus until it enters into the stomach. It is a complex process involving the muscular and neurological system. The mechanism of swallowing has been divided into three phases [1, 2]:

- Oral phase:
    - Oral preparatory phase
    - Oral propulsive phase
- Pharyngeal phase
- Esophageal phase

Variations may occur in the duration and characteristics of each of these phases with change in the food consistency and the amount of food consumed in a single swallow, as well as the age of a person and voluntary control on the swallowed bolus [3, 4]. Also, in a spontaneous swallow, as in swallowing saliva, the oral phase is bypassed in most cases [5].

G. Mankekar, MS, DNB, PhD (✉)
ENT, ex-PD Hinduja Hospital and AJBM ENT Hospital, Mahim, Mumbai, India
e-mail: gaurimankekar@gmail.com

K. Chavan, MBBS, DNB
ENT, Dr. L.H. Hiranandani Hospital, Powai, Mumbai, India
e-mail: kashuc@yahoo.com

© Springer India 2015
G. Mankekar (ed.), *Swallowing – Physiology, Disorders, Diagnosis and Therapy*,
DOI 10.1007/978-81-322-2419-8_2

Two models are commonly used to describe the physiology of normal eating and swallowing [1]:

- *The four-stage model* for drinking and swallowing liquids
- *The process model* for eating and swallowing solid food.

The normal swallow has been traditionally described with a three-stage sequential model, classified into oral, pharyngeal, and esophageal phases depending on the location of the food bolus in the swallowing passage. The oral phase was subsequently divided into oral preparatory and oral propulsive stages. This four-stage model describes swallowing of liquids adequately.

The process model was proposed as it was thought that the earlier model could not adequately describe the swallowing mechanism for solid food, especially food transport and bolus formation in the oropharynx [1, 6, 7].

After the food has been chewed and proper consistency achieved, it passes posteriorly for bolus formation in the oropharynx (including the valleculae), several seconds before the pharyngeal phase of a swallow. Some of the food can pass into the oropharynx and accumulate there while the remaining portion continues to be masticated in the oral cavity. Thus there is an overlap between the oral preparatory, oral propulsive, and pharyngeal phases.

Oral Phase

The oral phase of swallowing is composed of a sequence of events involving incising of food by the front teeth, transport of food towards the posterior teeth, mastication and chewing of the food into smaller pieces, and directing the food bolus towards the pharynx.

Oral Preparatory Phase [1, 8]

After liquid is taken into the mouth, the bolus is held between the anterior part of the floor of the mouth or tongue surface and the hard palate surrounded by the upper dental arch (Fig. 2.1a). The orbicularis oris contracts to seal the lips tightly. Jaw closure is brought about by the contraction of the masticatory muscles. Contraction of the buccinator keeps the cheek pressed against the teeth, keeping the cheek taut and preventing food from accumulating between the teeth and the cheek. The soft palate comes in contact with the posterior end of the tongue due to contraction of the palatoglossal and palatopharyngeal arches, sealing the oral cavity from the oropharynx, thus preventing entry of food into the oropharynx. The salivary glands secrete saliva into the oral cavity to convert the food into a bolus for

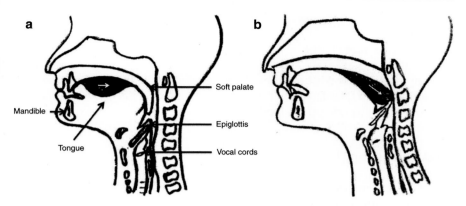

Fig. 2.1 Oral phase of swallowing: (**a**) the bolus is held between the anterior end of the tongue and the hard palate during the initiation of the oral phase and (**b**) the bolus is propelled into the pharynx to trigger the pharyngeal phase

swallowing. Tongue movements push the food onto the grinding surfaces of the teeth. The food is chewed and mixed with the salivary secretions to change its consistency to prepare it for the swallow. During this phase, breathing through the nose continues as the airway is open and the larynx and pharynx are at rest. Any weakness of the tongue or soft palate muscles can lead to leakage of food into the oropharynx during this phase.

Oral Propulsive Phase [1, 8]

During this stage, the tongue tip is raised by the action of the intrinsic muscles of the tongue and the genioglossus so that the tongue touches the alveolar ridge of the hard palate just posterior to the upper teeth. The posterior end of the tongue is depressed to open the posterior portion of the oral cavity. Elevation of the mandible helps in elevating the hyoid bone (brought about by the suprahyoid muscles) and the floor of the mouth. Simultaneously, the tongue surface also moves in the upward direction, so that the area of tongue–palate contact gradually increases from anterior to posterior and the liquid bolus is squeezed along the palate into the oropharynx. When the bolus reaches the posterior part of the tongue, the soft palate is elevated by the levator and tensor palatini muscles, sealing the nasopharynx from the oropharynx, thus preventing nasal regurgitation. Weakness of the palatal muscles or structural abnormalities like a cleft palate can lead to regurgitation of food into the nasopharynx and nasal cavity. When drinking liquids, the pharyngeal phase normally begins during oral propulsion (Fig. 2.1b).

Process Model of Feeding

Stage I Transport [1, 7]

Once ingested, the food is carried by tongue movements to the postcanine region. The tongue then rotates laterally. This places the food onto the occlusal surface of lower teeth for the next stage of food processing.

Food Processing [1, 7]

This is the next immediate stage after stage 1 transport. The food is broken down into smaller particles by chewing and softened by salivary secretions to achieve a proper consistency to make it ready for bolus formation and swallow. Chewing continues until all of the food is prepared. As opposed to the oral preparatory phase during drinking of liquids, there is no sealing of the posterior oral cavity from the pharynx by contact of the posterior tongue with the soft palate during food processing. During food processing, cyclic movements of the tongue, soft palate, and jaw lead to an open passage between the oral cavity and pharynx. Food aroma reaches the nasal chemoreceptors by pumping of air into the nasal cavity by tongue and jaw movements. Vertical, mediolateral, and rotational tongue movements along with coordinated jaw and cheek movements keep the food on the occlusal surfaces of the lower teeth. Forward and downward movement of the tongue, during early to mid jaw opening, followed by backward movement of the tongue during late jaw opening prevents tongue bites during a normal swallow. Movement of the hyoid bone by its muscular attachments also controls the tongue and jaw mobility. Any weakness of the tongue, jaw, or cheek musculature can interfere with this stage.

Stage II Transport [1, 7]

Stage II transport is similar to the oral propulsive stage with a liquid bolus. The anterior end of the tongue comes into contact with the hard palate just behind the upper incisors. The area of tongue–palate contact gradually expands antero-posteriorly, squeezing the processed food posteriorly along the palate to the oropharynx. Stage II transport primarily occurs secondary to tongue movements and does not require gravity. The transported food accumulates on the pharyngeal surface of the tongue and in the valleculae, while the food remaining in the oral cavity is chewed and the size of the bolus in the oropharynx progressively enlarges. In normal individuals, the duration of bolus aggregation in the oropharynx while eating solid food varies from a fraction of a second to about 10 s [1, 7].

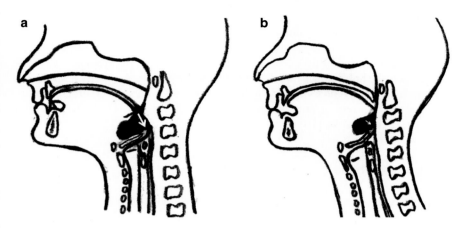

Fig. 2.2 Pharyngeal phase of swallow: the soft palate is elevated and in contact with the pharyngeal wall. The laryngeal inlet is protected by the epiglottis. (**a**) Bolus in the vallecula and (**b**) the tongue base retracted posteriorly towards the pharyngeal wall

Pharyngeal Phase

This phase is composed of a series of sequential events for the passage of the food bolus from the pharynx to the esophagus along with protection of the airway and nasopharynx (Fig. 2.2).

The passage of food bolus through the fauces was earlier thought to act as a sensory input to trigger the initiation of the pharyngeal stage [1, 9, 10]. The sensory input for the initiation of this reflex is carried by the vagus and the glossopharyngeal nerves to the swallowing center in the brainstem [10]. Variable bolus position at swallow initiation has been demonstrated by various studies, which have shown that bolus entry into the pharynx may occur before swallow initiation in healthy individuals when drinking liquids [1, 11, 12]. Food may enter the hypopharynx before a swallow, especially in case of food that contains both solid and liquid components [1]. Thus the trigger for swallow initiation may depend on multiple factors [12]. Also while eating solid food, the chewed bolus is aggregated in the oropharynx or valleculae before swallowing.

When the bolus enters the oropharynx, the nasopharynx is closed by elevation and contact of the soft palate with the lateral and posterior pharyngeal walls, thus preventing nasal regurgitation. This velopharyngeal closure, brought about by the levator palatine muscles also provides a surface to propel the bolus in a downward direction. The velopharyngeal closure is shortly followed by reflex closure of the laryngeal inlet. Closure of the true and false vocal cords occurs. The hyoid bone and larynx are pulled upward and forward due to suprahyoid and thyrohyoid muscle contraction, so that the larynx is covered by the tongue base [1, 7, 8, 10]. Backward movement of the epiglottis, probably thought to be due to hyolaryngeal elevation, pharyngeal constriction, bolus movement, and tongue base retraction covers the laryngeal inlet [13]. This results in apnea which may last from 0.5 to 1.5 s [1, 14, 15]. Retraction of the base tongue pushes the bolus against the pharyngeal walls. Sequential contraction of the constrictor muscles of the pharynx from above downward propels the bolus downward. The volume of the pharyngeal cavity reduces due to decrease in vertical pharyngeal length. The constrictor muscles contract involuntarily, but their actions are coordinated via the pharyngeal plexus [10]. The duration of this phase is about 1 s [10].

Esophageal Phase

The esophageal phase begins when the food bolus enters the esophagus. The esophagus is made up of smooth and striated muscle and is innervated by the esophageal plexus of nerves. The upper esophageal sphincter (UES) is in a state of constant contraction [16]. The UES opens up to allow the passage of the food bolus into the esophagus. Impaired UES opening can lead to food retention in the piriform sinuses and hypopharynx, increasing the risk of aspiration following a swallow. Factors responsible for the opening of the UES are [1]:

• Cricopharyngeus muscle relaxation (usually prior to the arrival of the food bolus and UES opening)
• Suprahyoid and thyrohyoid muscle contraction, which results in an anterior pull on the hyoid bone and the larynx, thus opening the UES
• Mechanical pressure offered by the bolus

The lower esophageal sphincter, which is also contracted at rest [16] (which helps in prevention of gastric reflux), relaxes when the food bolus reaches it. The bolus is transported by a peristaltic wave through the lower esophageal sphincter into the stomach [10]. The peristalsis in the thoracic esophagus is "true peristalsis" regulated by the autonomic nervous system [1]. The peristaltic wave consists of an initial wave of relaxation that accommodates the bolus, followed by a wave of contraction that propels it [1]. This is further assisted by gravity when in an upright position [1]. During this phase, the soft palate is lowered by the relaxation of the tensor and levator palatine muscles, the hyoid drops down, the epiglottis goes back to its original position, and the laryngeal vestibule opens [8] (Fig. 2.3).

A normal swallow requires coordination between mastication, respiration, and swallowing [1, 8, 10]. The process of swallowing is partially voluntary and partly involuntary. Centers in the brain are responsible for the voluntary control of swallowing. Bilateral areas in the primary sensory and motor cortex, in the prefrontal areas (anterior to the face region of the precentral gyrus, corresponding to Brodmann area 6), and in the parietal cortex are related to the voluntary initiation of swallowing [8]. The control of swallowing in humans is complex, with some areas being controlled bilaterally, while others are under unilateral control [8].

In addition to the mechanical sealing of the larynx during the pharyngeal phase of swallowing, respiration is also interrupted by the inhibition of the respiratory

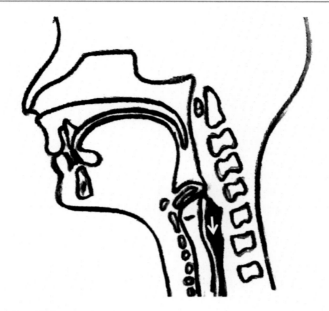

Fig. 2.3 Esophageal phase

center in the brainstem [1, 17]. Swallowing of a liquid usually starts at the expiratory phase of respiration, and completion of swallow is followed by resumption of respiration in the expiratory phase. This acts as a protective mechanism, as it helps in clearing out any residues, thus preventing aspiration [1, 14, 15]. The respiratory rhythm is also altered during mastication of solid food. During swallowing of solid food, the apneic phase may be slightly longer [1].

The physiology of swallowing is a complex process involving coordination between various systems. Any abnormality in the swallowing pathway, anatomical or neural, can lead to swallowing dysfunction. Also, central neurological disorders can affect swallowing in the presence of an anatomically normal swallowing pathway. Aspiration pneumonia, malnutrition, etc., are some of the consequences of swallowing disorders. A detailed understanding of the factors controlling the swallowing mechanism with respect to its structure and neural control would help in diagnosing and treating swallowing disorders.

Esophageal Function Tests

Introduction

Swallowing disorders may be due to numerous causes ranging from intrinsic, intramural, to extrinsic and motility disorders of the esophagus. A battery of tests may be required to diagnose esophageal causes of dysphagia. These tests include esophageal manometry, fiberoptic endoscopic evaluation of swallowing, and esophageal ultrasound.

Esophageal Manometry

Esophageal manometry is used to measure the amplitude and coordination of esophageal muscle contraction and relaxation and activity of the upper and lower esophageal sphincters.

Indications [18]
- Evaluation of nonobstructive dysphagia, especially when achalasia is suspected
- During placement of intraluminal devices (e.g., pH probes) to accurately localize the lower esophageal sphincter for correct probe positioning
- Preoperative assessment of patients being considered for antireflux surgery, if an alternative diagnosis, like achalasia, is being considered
- Preoperative assessment of peristalsis in patients scheduled for antireflux surgery
- Postoperative evaluation of dysphagia in patients who have undergone antireflux surgery or achalasia treatment

Contraindications
- Esophageal manometry is not indicated for making or confirming a suspected diagnosis of gastroesophageal reflux disease.
- It should not be routinely used as the initial test for chest pain or other esophageal symptoms.
- Suspected or known obstructive pathology (e.g., tumors).
- Uncooperative patients.
- Bleeding/clotting disorders.

Equipment
The components of the manometry system are:

- Esophageal manometry catheter (water perfusion or solid state)
- Pressure transducers
- Signal acquisition
- Information storage devices (software, computer)
- Lidocaine spray, viscous lidocaine, tapes, lubricating gel, syringes, etc.

The esophageal manometry catheter is a long, flexible tube that is placed in the patient's esophagus with the distal tip lying in the stomach. The catheters can be made of a variety of plastic materials, most frequently polyvinyl chloride or silicone. The tip is slightly curved and may include a weighted distal metal tip to facilitate passage into the stomach.

The patient should not have anything to eat or drink at least 4 h prior to the procedure (diabetic patients should be NPO past midnight the night prior to the procedure). Regular medications can be taken with a small amount of water. While some medications may alter esophageal motility (e.g., antispasmodics, prokinetic agents, analgesics, sedatives), if the patient is taking them on a daily basis for a chronic condition, it makes sense to perform the study while the patient is on these medications, so as to factor in their systemic effects in the test results and decide on possible further therapy.

Pre-procedure Requirements
The patient should be nil by mouth for at least 4–6 h prior to the procedure. Regular medications can be taken with a small amount of water. Medications like calcium channel blockers, sedatives, antispasmodics, prokinetics, analgesics, etc., that may alter esophageal motility should be discontinued 24 h prior to the procedure. However if the patient has been taking these drugs on a long-term basis for certain chronic conditions, sometimes performing the test while the patient is on these medications may help in considering their effects on esophageal function so as to decide the further course of therapy.

Anesthesia
Topical anesthesia with lidocaine spray and viscous lidocaine.

Procedure
Lubricating jelly is applied to the tip of the catheter. A few minutes after the topical anesthesia is administered, with the patient in upright sitting position, the catheter is passed transnasally. The catheter will be at the level of the hypopharynx when about 12 cm of the length is passed. The patient is then asked to take small sips of water so as to relax the lower esophageal sphincter (LES) and the catheter is slowly advanced further. The most distal transducer will show rise in pressure as the catheter passes the LES. The patient is then made supine and gastric baseline pressures are measured when the catheter enters the stomach. The patient is asked to take a deep breath. Intra-abdominal pressure readings go up with inspiration and decrease on expiration. The catheter is then slowly withdrawn, watching for increase in pressures, indicating its position at the LES.

Once the distal most transducer is in the LES, ten 5 ml water swallows are given to the patient at intervals of 20–30 s to evaluate the LES relaxation pattern and contraction of the distal esophageal smooth muscle. The catheter is then pulled out, 0.5 cm at a time, allowing the patient to take a few breaths between moves without swallowing. The proximal border of the LES is identified when the pressure pattern shows decrease with inspiration and increase on expiration indicating the thoracic position of the transducer. Once the area of maximal upper esophageal sphincter (UES) pressure is reached, the catheter is manipulated to place the most proximal transducer 1 cm below the UES. Five 5 ml water swallows are then administered to evaluate the contraction pattern of the proximal esophageal muscle.

The patient is then placed in an upright sitting position to evaluate the UES and the pharynx. The catheter is withdrawn slowly until the distal transducer is located at the UES with a drop in pressure when the transducer reaches the proximal portion of the UES. Six 5 ml water swallows are then administered. An M-shaped pressure configuration pattern is usually noticed at this time with each swallow as the UES elevates onto the transducer (first pressure spike), then relaxes (first pressure fall), closes (second pressure spike), and finally descends onto its original position (second pressure fall).

High-resolution manometry (HRM) is being used in recent times [19]. Conventional manometry requires multiple maneuvers to reposition the catheter at the LES. With HRM, there is no need to move the catheter as the 36-channeled catheter occupies the entire esophagus simultaneously. The UES, LES, and the rest of the esophagus can be assessed simultaneously with a single series of swallows with the catheter in a single, fixed position. As the channels in the conventional water-perfused catheters are widely spaced, findings may be missed at times. The water-perfused catheters are stationary at the LES; hence, during swallows, esophageal shortening may lead to proximal LES displacement, giving a false interpretation of LES relaxation. HRM gives color contours as against waveforms seen with conventional manometry. HRM catheters are less stiff and the technique is less cumbersome and quicker (as multiple manipulations and pull-through techniques are not required) [19].

Complications
Mild complications such as gagging due to inadequate topical anesthesia or a strong gag reflex, rhinorrhea, and epistaxis (due to traumatic catheter insertion).

Rare Complications
- Vasovagal episodes
- Arrhythmias
- Bronchospasm aspiration
- Esophageal perforation [20]

Interpretation

The Chicago Classification classifies esophageal motility disorders based on HRM findings (Table 2.1) [21]:

- PFV: Pressurization front velocity (PFV), calculated from the 30 mmHg isobaric contour plots by marking the distal temporal margin of the transition zone and the superior margin of the EGJ on the 30 mmHg isobaric contour and then calculating the slope between the two, expressed in cm/s. A normal PFV depends upon both an intact distal peristaltic contraction and normal EGJ relaxation.
- DCI: Distal esophageal contraction was characterized for the vigor of contraction using the distal contractile integral (DCI). The DCI quantifies the length, vigor, and persistence of postdeglutitive pressurization in the distal esophageal segment, expressed as mmHg-s-cm.
- EGJ: Esophagogastric junction.

Table 2.1 Esophageal motility classification on the basis of pressure topography criteria (the Chicago Classification) [21]

Normal
PFV <8 cm/s in >90 % of swallows
DCI <5,000 mmHg-s-cm
Normal EGJ pressure (10–35 mmHg) and deglutitive relaxation (eSleeve 3 s nadir <15 mmHg)
Peristaltic dysfunction
Mild: either ≥3 and <7 swallows with failed peristalsis or a ≥2 cm defect in the 30 mmHg isobaric contour of the distal esophageal segment
Severe: either ≥7 swallows with failed peristalsis or a ≥2 cm defect in the 30 mmHg isobaric contour of the distal esophageal segment
Aperistalsis
No continuous pressure domain above an isobaric contour of 30 mmHg in the distal esophageal segment in any swallow
Scleroderma pattern: no continuous pressure domain above an isobaric contour of 30 mmHg in the distal esophageal segment in any swallow and a mean LES pressure <10 mmHg
Hypertensive peristalsis
PFV <8 cm/s in >90 % of swallows
Mean DCI: >5,000 mmHg-s-cm
Nutcracker: mean DCI >5,000 and <8,000 mmHg-s-cm
Segmental nutcracker: mean DCI >5,000 with only one segmental focus of hypertensive contraction (>180 mmHg)
Spastic nutcracker: mean DCI >8,000 mmHg-s-cm
Nutcracker LES: mean DCI >5,000 mmHg-s-cm with the focus of hypertensive contraction (>180 mmHg) limited to the LES after-contraction
Rapidly propagated pressurization
PFV >8 cm/s in ≥20 % of swallows
Spasm (increased PFV attributable to rapid contractile wavefront)
Compartmentalized pressurization (increased PFV attributable to distal compartmentalized esophageal pressurization)
Abnormal LES tone (end expiratory)
Hypotensive: mean <10 mmHg with normal peristaltic function
Hypertensive: mean >35 mmHg with normal peristaltic function and EGJ relaxation
Achalasia
Impaired deglutitive EGJ relaxation
Aperistalsis
Classic: aperistalsis or panesophageal pressurization with no identifiable segmental contractile activity with all swallows
Vigorous: with distal spasm
Functional obstruction
Impaired deglutitive EGJ relaxation
Mild: PFV <8 cm/s in >90 % of swallows with a mild elevation (15–30 mmHg) of distal esophageal pressurization
Severe: PFV >8 cm/s in ≥20 % of swallows with compartmentalized pressurization

Flexible Endoscopic Evaluation of Swallowing (FEES)

Flexible endoscopic evaluation of swallowing (FEES) is a procedure to endoscopically examine the pharyngeal stage of swallow using a flexible endoscope. It allows the evaluation of the laryngopharyngeal anatomy and physiology during a swallow. FEES when combined with sensory testing is called FEESST (flexible endoscopic evaluation of swallowing with sensory testing) and is used to evaluate laryngeal sensations.

Indications [22]

- Assessing secretions and their management
- Evaluation of patients at high risk of aspiration
- Direct visualization and assessment of laryngopharyngeal anatomy
- Biofeedback/teaching during swallow therapy
- Assessment of therapeutic interventions
- Assessing swallow fatigue
- Assessment of swallowing of specific foods
- In patients unable to undergo videofluoroscopy
- Patients in whom repeated assessments may be required

Equipment

- Flexible nasolaryngoscope (with a side channel if FEESST is to be performed, for delivery of air pulse stimulus)
- Light source
- Video equipment (camera, monitor)
- Calibrated air pulse sensory stimulator (for FEESST)

Anesthesia

Although it is feared that a topical anesthesia spray through the nose may interfere with laryngeal or pharyngeal function, some authors have reported no obvious motion abnormalities with the use of topical anesthesia. Most studies however do not advocate the use of topical anesthesia. A nasal decongestant such as topical oxymetazoline may be used.

Procedure

FEES is usually performed by an otolaryngologist along with a speech–language pathologist. The patient should be awake in an unreclined, seated position. The flexible nasolaryngoscope is introduced transnasally. As the scope is passed, all the structures including the nasopharynx, soft palate, base tongue, valleculae, epiglottis, arytenoids, aryepiglottic folds, pyriform fossae, vocal cords, and the postcricoid region are evaluated. The pharyngeal squeeze maneuver is performed first. During this maneuver, the patient is asked to make high-pitched, strained phonation (high-pitched e) and pharyngeal squeeze is observed. A good pharyngeal squeeze is an indication of good pharyngeal musculature strength and swallowing safety [23]. The patient is then asked to begin oral intake, starting with sips of water, followed by thin liquids, thick liquids, puree, soft food, solid food, and mixed consistencies. The amount of premature spillage, residue in the valleculae or hypopharynx, laryngeal penetration (bolus entering the laryngeal inlet), and laryngeal aspiration (bolus going past the laryngeal inlet) are observed. A quick look at the trachea may be performed if possible to confirm aspiration. The initiation of the swallow, strength of swallow, fatigue, timing, and adequacy of glottic closure and regurgitation are also looked for. In order to perform FEESST, an air puff stimulus is delivered to the laryngeal mucosa innervated by the superior laryngeal nerve on both the right side and left side to elicit a laryngeal adductor reflex (LAR) [24, 25].

The flexible laryngoscope is placed above the junction of the arytenoid and aryepiglottic fold junction and graded air puff stimuli are delivered. Laryngopharyngeal sensory discrimination thresholds are defined as [25]:

- Normal: <4 mmHg air pulse pressure
- Moderate: 4–6 mmHg air pulse pressure
- Severe: >6.0 mmHg air pulse pressure

The presence of bilateral deficits indicates poor swallowing [23].

Complications [22]

Complications are rare during this procedure. Some of the difficulties that may be encountered are:

- Patient discomfort
- Epistaxis: due to trauma during endoscope introduction
- Vasovagal response
- Reflex syncope
- Allergy to topical anesthesia
- Laryngospasm (rare)

Transnasal Esophagoscopy (TNE)

Transnasal esophagoscopy (TNE) is an in-office procedure used in the diagnosis of esophageal disorders as well as to perform additional interventional procedures. Unlike traditional upper gastrointestinal endoscopy, it does not require sedation and has been found to be an efficient and safe procedure.

Indications [26]

Esophageal
- Dysphagia
- Refractory gastroesophageal reflux disease
- Screening for Barrett's esophagus/carcinoma

Extra-esophageal
- Significant globus
- Screening for head and neck cancer
- Moderate to severe EER chronic cough

Procedure Related
- Panendoscopy for head and neck cancer
- Biopsy
- Botox injection
- Balloon dilation
- Percutaneous endoscopic gastrostomy
- Tracheoesophageal puncture
- Placement of wireless pH monitoring device (capsules)

Contraindications

There are no absolute contraindications to TNE.

Relative Contraindications
- Presence of diverticula
- Coagulation disorders
- Uncooperative patient

Equipment
Transnasal endoscopes are usually longer and thinner (3.1–5.1 mm) than conventional endoscopes. A working channel is provided to pass instruments (e.g., biopsy forceps).

Pre-procedure Requirements

The procedure is performed as an in-office procedure. The patient should be nil by mouth for about 3–4 h before the procedure. The patient is in a sitting position. Vital signs should be recorded at the beginning of the procedure.

Anesthesia

Adequate topical nasal anesthesia and nasal decongestion are obtained. A local lignocaine spray is also administered to the oropharynx. Viscous lidocaine may also be used. However, excessive local anesthesia may cause pooling of secretions.

Technique

The endoscope is lubricated and passed transnasally into the nasopharynx. It is then gradually advanced further to visualize the larynx and hypopharynx. The patient is asked to flex the head and the endoscope position is maintained just superior to the postcricoid region. The patient is then asked to perform swallowing movements so that the scope is gently introduced into the esophagus. The lumen is kept in sight at all times as the scope is advanced up to the LES with gentle air insufflation and suctioning. The esophageal motility is evaluated as the patient swallows. Just when the scope is proximal to the LES, the LES function is evaluated (whether the LES is closed at rest, if it opens, and immediately closes after swallowing). The scope is then advanced into the stomach and retroflexion performed (by rotating the entire endoscope 180° and maximally deflecting the endoscope tip 210°) to visualize the gastroesophageal junction and cardia of the stomach. Extra air may be required for adequate visualization. Additional air is suctioned out to prevent abdominal discomfort before the scope is slowly withdrawn. Sampling of lesions can be performed by passing biopsy forceps through the working channel of the scope.

Complications

Complications occurring with TNE are rare. Epistaxis or vasovagal syncope can occur very rarely [26]. One case of perforation following TNE performed by a gastroenterologist has been reported [27].

Esophageal Ultrasound

Endoscopic ultrasound is a procedure used to diagnose and treat a variety of gastrointestinal lesions. Endoscopic ultrasound of the esophagus can be utilized to visualize mucosal, submucosal, and extraluminal esophageal pathologies.

Standard echoendoscopes use ultrasound frequencies ranging from 5 to 12 MHz which enable tissue imaging up to 5–6 cm depth from the transducer but at a relatively low resolution [28]. Catheter ultrasound probes or miniprobes, which are passed through the side channel of standard endoscopes, use frequencies between 7.5 and 20 MHz and enable imaging of tissues at a depth of 1–2 cm from the transducer at a higher resolution [28].

Indications [28, 29]

- To differentiate between benign and malignant esophageal pathologies.
- To differentiate between submucosal and extraluminal pathologies. An upper gastrointestinal endoscopy may reveal a bulge in the esophageal wall but may not be able to clearly define if the bulge is due to a submucosal lesion or an extraluminal compressive pathology.
- To define the extent and invasion of lesions and nodal staging in esophageal cancers.
- To carry out endoscopic ultrasound-guided fine-needle aspiration biopsy.
- To rule out underlying malignancy in motility disorders (secondary achalasia).
- Cytologic sampling of nonesophageal tumors (e.g. lymph nodes in lung carcinoma).

Contraindications

Contraindications to an endoscopic esophageal ultrasound are the same as those for a routine endoscopy such as a suspected perforation and uncooperative patient. Fine needle aspiration of lesions distal to a stricture may be a relative contra indication. The fine needle aspiration may be performed after dilating the stricture.

Technique

The procedure is performed under sedation similar to a routine esophagoscopy. A regular endoscopy is performed first to look at the anatomy and any obvious abnormalities in the esophageal lining. The endoscope is then withdrawn and an ultrasound scope passed in a similar manner. Smaller ultrasound probes are also available which can be passed through a side channel in the standard scope. Fine-needle aspiration can be performed in the same sitting if indicated. Five layers are visualized on esophageal echoendoscopy, corresponding to the histologic layers of the esophagus [30]:

- *The innermost layer* (*lumen*): hyperechoic or echogenic, due to the interface between the ultrasound waves, the gastrointestinal tract mucosa, and surrounding fluid.
- *Second layer*: hypoechoic or dark band corresponding to the mucosa and deep mucosa

- *Third layer*: hyperechoic or bright echo corresponding to the submucosa
- *Fourth layer*: hypoechoic or dark band corresponding to the muscularis propria
- *Fifth layer*: hyperechoic or bright echogenic band corresponding to the adventitia

In addition to these, the four more layers are visualized when a high-frequency probe is used [31]. These layers correspond to the following:

- Superficial epithelium
- Deep epithelium
- Lamina propria plus the acoustic interface echo between the lamina propria and muscularis mucosa
- Muscularis mucosa minus the acoustic interface echo between the lamina propria and muscularis mucosa

Complications

Complications of endoscopic esophageal ultrasound are similar to those associated with an upper GI endoscopy and include:

- Pain
- Hemorrhage
- Perforation
- Infection

The abovementioned esophageal function tests are a helpful tool to the clinician in reaching an accurate diagnosis in the case of esophageal disorders.

References

1. Palmer JB, Matsuo K. Anatomy and physiology of feeding and swallowing: normal and abnormal. Phys Med Rehabil Clin N Am. 2008;19:691–707.
2. Shaker R, Belafsky PC, Postma GN. Caryn Easterling principles of deglutition: a multidisciplinary text for swallowing and its disorders. New York: Springer; 2013.
3. Mendell DA, Logemann JA. Temporal sequence of swallow events during the oropharyngeal swallow. J Speech Lang Hear Res. 2007;50(5):1256–71.
4. Kahrilas PJ, Logemann JA. Volume accommodation during swallowing. Dysphagia. 1993;8(3):259–65.
5. Ertekin C. Voluntary versus spontaneous swallowing in man. Dysphagia. 2011;26(2):183–92.
6. Palmer JB, Rudin NJ, Lara G, et al. Coordination of mastication and swallowing. Dysphagia. 1992;7(4):187–200.
7. Hiiemae KM, Palmer JB. Food transport and bolus formation during complete feeding sequences on foods of different initial consistency. Dysphagia. 1999;14(1):31–42.
8. Gleeson M, Browning GG, Burton MJ, Clarke R, John H, Jones NS, Lund VJ, Luxon LM, Watkinson JC. Scott-Brown's otorhinolaryngology, head and neck surgery. 7th ed. London: Hodder Arnold; 2008.

9. Logemann JA. Evaluation and treatment of swallowing disorders. 2nd ed. Austin: Pro-Ed; 1998.
10. Merati A, Bielamowicz S, editors. Textbook of laryngology. San Diego: Plural Publishing; 2006.
11. Martin-Harris B, Brodsky MB, Michel Y, et al. Delayed initiation of the pharyngeal swallow: normal variability in adult swallows. J Speech Lang Hear Res. 2007;50(3):585–94.
12. Stephen JR, Taves DH, Smith RC, et al. Bolus location at the initiation of the pharyngeal stage of swallowing in healthy older adults. Dysphagia. 2005;20(4):266–72.
13. Logemann JA, Kahrilas PJ, Cheng J, et al. Closure mechanisms of laryngeal vestibule during swallow. Am J Physiol. 1992;262(2 Pt 1):G338–44.
14. Selley WG, Flack FC, Ellis RE, et al. Respiratory patterns associated with swallowing: part 1. The normal adult pattern and changes with age. Age Ageing. 1989;18(3):168–72.
15. Klahn MS, Perlman AL. Temporal and durational patterns associating respiration and swallowing. Dysphagia. 1999;14(3):131–8.
16. Bailey BJ, Johnson JT, Newlands SD. Head & neck surgery–otolaryngology, vol. 1. Philadelphia: Lippincott Williams and Wilkins; 1993.
17. Nishino T, Hiraga K. Coordination of swallowing and respiration in unconscious subjects. J Appl Physiol. 1991;70(3):988–93.
18. Pandolfino JE, Kahrilas PJ, American Gastroenterological Association. American Gastroenterological Association medical position statement: clinical use of esophageal manometry. Gastroenterology. 2005;128(1):207–8.
19. Conklin J, Pimentel M, Soffer E, editors. Esophageal manometry. Color atlas of high resolution manometry. New York: Springer; 2009.
20. Meister V, Schulz H, Greving I, et al. Perforation of the esophagus after esophageal manometry. Dtsch Med Wochenschr. 1997;122(46):1410–4.
21. Kahrilas PJ, Ghosh SK, Pandolfino JE. Esophageal motility disorders in terms of pressure topography: the Chicago classification. J Clin Gastroenterol. 2008;42(5):627–35.
22. Kelly AM, Hydes K, McLaughlin C, Wallace S. Fibreoptic Endoscopic Evaluation of Swallowing (FEES): the role of speech and language therapy. Royal College of Speech and Language Therapists. Policy Statement 2005. Advised review date 2007. http://www.sld.cu/galerias/pdf/sitios/rehabilitacion-logo/evaluacion_endoscopica_de_la_deglucion.pdf.
23. Merati LA. In-office evaluation of swallowing FEES, pharyngeal squeeze maneuver, and FEESST. Otolaryngol Clin N Am. 2013;46:31–9.
24. Aviv JE, Martin JH, Keen MS, et al. Air pulse quantification of supraglottic and pharyngeal sensation: a new technique. Ann Otol Rhinol Laryngol. 1993;102(10):777–80.
25. Aviv JE, Kim T, Sacco RL, et al. FEESST: a new bedside endoscopic test of the motor and sensory components of swallowing. Ann Otol Rhinol Laryngol. 1998;107(5 Pt 1):378–87.
26. Bush CM, Postma GM. Transnasal esophagoscopy. Otolaryngol Clin N Am. 2013;46:41–52.
27. Zaman A, Hahn M, Hapke R, et al. A randomized trial of peroral versus transnasal unsedated endoscopy using an ultrathin videoendoscope. Gastrointest Endosc. 1999;49:279–84.
28. Byrne MF, Jowell PS. Gastrointestinal imaging: endoscopic ultrasound. Gastroenterology. 2002;122:1631–48.
29. Trindade AJ, Berzin TM. Clinical controversies in endoscopic ultrasound. Gastroenterol Rep (Oxf). 2013;1(1):33–41.
30. Kimmey MB, Martin RW, Haggitt RC, et al. Histologic correlates of gastrointestinal ultrasound images. Gastroenterology. 1989;96(2 Pt 1):433.
31. Wiersema MJ, Wiersema LM. High-resolution 25-megahertz ultrasonography of the gastrointestinal wall: histologic correlates. Gastrointest Endosc. 1993;39(4):499.

Dysphagia: Clinical Diagnosis

3

Gauri Mankekar

Introduction

Dysphagia or difficulty in swallowing can present either as food getting stuck or as coughing spells during swallowing. The diagnosis of dysphagia could be done by a physician, an otolaryngologist, a pulmonologist, and an intensive care specialist who has recently extubated a patient, or it could be a gastroenterologist or a neurologist or even an oncologist treating head-neck cancers. The consequences of dysphagia can range from malnutrition, dehydration, to persistent cough or aspiration pneumonia. Therefore, it is imperative to identify the cause of dysphagia and treat the patient. As with all medical conditions, the diagnosis of dysphagia starts with taking a thorough history, followed by examination and specific tests.

History

The patient's description and duration of their dysphagia often helps to point towards the cause of the swallowing problem:

1. *Onset*: Sudden onset of dysphagia, especially in children and in the elderly, could mean foreign body impaction. Onset following extubation for either general anesthesia or mechanical ventilation could suggest oropharyngeal-laryngeal injury during intubation/extubation or supraglottic or arytenoid edema.
2. *Duration:* Short duration of swallowing difficulty often indicates either a foreign body obstruction or an inflammation secondary to candidiasis or CMV infection or eosinophilic esophagitis. Rapid progression (weeks or months) of dysphagia

G. Mankekar, MS, DNB, PhD
ENT, ex-PD Hinduja Hospital and AJBM ENT Hospital, Mahim, Mumbai, India
e-mail: gaurimankekar@gmail.com

© Springer India 2015
G. Mankekar (ed.), *Swallowing – Physiology, Disorders, Diagnosis and Therapy*,
DOI 10.1007/978-81-322-2419-8_3

39

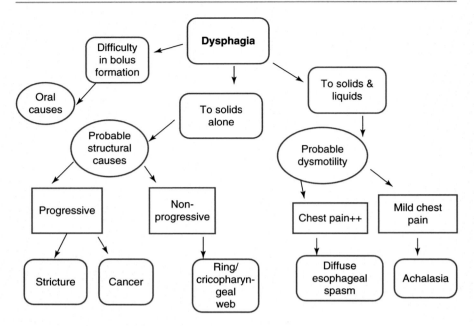

Fig. 3.1 Algorithm for clinical diagnosis of dysphagia

with associated weight loss could suggest esophageal malignancy. On the other hand, long-standing, intermittent, non-progressive dysphagia mainly for solids is suggestive of a structural lesion like a distal esophageal ring or proximal esophageal mucosal web [1]. If the dysphagia has been long standing and slowly progressive associated with gastroesophageal reflux, then it could suggest a peptic stricture. But the severity of heartburn correlates poorly with the degree of esophageal mucosal damage [2].

3. *Type*: (Fig. 3.1) Edentulous patients will describe swallowing difficulty and coughing spells during intake of solid food. This is due to improper bolus formation during the oral phase of swallowing. Patients with motor disorders like achalasia or diffuse esophageal spasm describe dysphagia for liquids and solids, whereas patients with structural disorders complain about dysphagia for solids only [3]. However, dysphagia gets worse as solids obstruct the lumen. Hence, it is important to phrase the question properly when eliciting history of type of dysphagia as patients report dysphagia to both solids and liquids following impaction of a solid bolus irrespective of the underlying pathology.

4. *Associated symptoms*: Does patient cough or get chest pain associated with dysphagia? Dysphagia (for solids and liquids) with chest pain and regurgitation are the cardinal symptoms of esophageal motility disorders [4]. Regurgitation with foul smell is an indication of a pharyngeal diverticulum. In regurgitation associated with esophageal dysmotility, there is no foul smell.

Chest pain is associated with diffuse esophageal spasm or achalasia. It can be difficult to distinguish this "crushing" type of chest from that of the typical "heartburn" of reflux [5]. This pain often occurs during meals but can also be nocturnal and sporadic. Chest pain is often a prominent symptom in patients with early achalasia but decreases over the years as dysphagia and regurgitation worsen [6]. On the other hand, chest pain associated with esophageal spasm is severe and predominant, but regurgitation is not a prominent symptom.

Dysphagia in a scleroderma patient suggests a stricture as they mainly have reflux and regurgitation in the early stages.

If the bolus is obstructed at the cricopharyngeal sphincter level, then the patient could have coughing due to aspiration.

Pain associated with swallowing is called odynophagia. It may be due to oropharyngeal ulcers, tonsillopharyngitis, inflammation of the lingual tonsils, or even arytenoid inflammation.

Globus pharyngis is a sensation of either phlegm or something being stuck in the throat although no obstruction is actually found. These patients may develop the habit of continuously clearing their throat. They can swallow normally, and hence globus is not true dysphagia. Globus could be either psychogenic or due to inflammation of pharyngeal or laryngeal mucosa or gastroesophageal reflux.

5. How is dysphagia relieved? Does the patient drink water to relieve dysphagia? Sipping water often relieves dysphagia due to the bolus being held by a structural obstruction.

6. Associated history of medication intake: Prolonged use of proton pump inhibitors could suggest gastroesophageal reflux with Barrett's esophagus associated history of surgery/intubation – could suggest intubation trauma to soft palate, post pharyngeal wall, arytenoids, or postintubation pharyngeal or arytenoid edema causing dysphagia.

Physical Examination

General Examination

- *Age:* Young children may routinely have a certain amount of aspiration. However, the quantities are small and relatively quickly cleared from the lungs due to normal lung physiology and the normal immunological mechanisms especially as children are active and mobile. Persons over age 60 may have age-related changes in sensory discrimination of the tongue with reduced sensitivity (on tests of two-point discrimination) in the anterior two thirds of the tongue compared to people under 40 years [7]. Age-related changes in tongue motor function lead to prolonged oral transit time in individuals over 60 years of age when compared to people less than 60 [8]. An elderly patient complaining of a sensation of food (solids or liquids) sticking in his lower chest area with slight weight loss is likely to have achalasia. A middle-aged man with occasional dysphagia, who otherwise feels well and whose esophageal motility studies show an LES amplitude of approximately 60 mmHg and his esophagus relaxes completely when he swallows, is most likely to have hypertensive LES.

Fig. 3.2 Cervical
osteophytes (*arrow*)
impinging on
pharyngolaryngeal lumen

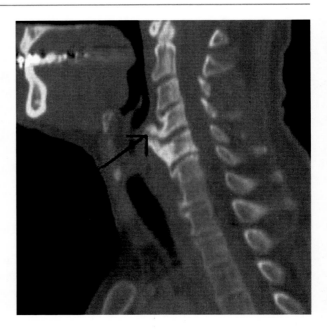

- *Appearance:* Cachexia in a patient with dysphagia could signify inadequate nutrition and therefore significant obstruction or immunocompromise.
  Immunocompromised patients have a reduced ability to fend off infection from normal or dysphagic aspiration. For other patients, the disease process may specifically affect the swallowing function.
- *Neurological:*
  - Testing cranial nerves V, VII, IX, X, and XII and evaluating movements of the mandible, muscles of mastication, facial muscles, tongue, and palate along with an assessment of the mass, strength, symmetry, and range of movement of the muscles. Facial nerve palsy can affect lip movements, leading to dribbling and therefore affecting the oral phase of swallowing.
  - Cough reflex. Loss of the cough reflex indicates decreased airway clearance, and these patients may have dysphonia with a "wet" or "bubbling" voice.
  - Complete neurological examination: Evaluating for cerebellar lesions (Wallenberg's syndrome), amyotrophic lateral sclerosis, etc.
- *Cervical movement:* It is imperative to check cervical movements in elderly patients with dysphagia. Radiological examination (plain X-ray neck lateral view or computed tomography scan) may show excess bone growths or osteophytes from the anterior part of the cervical spine impinging on the pharynx or esophagus leading to dysphagia (Fig. 3.2). Degenerative changes of the spine lead to formation of osteophytes. Occasionally, the condition may be a part of a disorder called diffuse idiopathic skeletal hyperostosis. Treatment can vary from observation to surgical removal of the osteophytes depending upon the severity of the symptoms.

Fig. 3.3 Edentulous patient

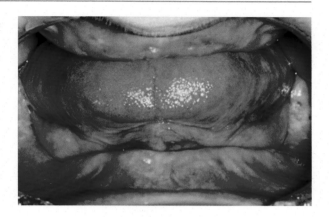

Fig. 3.4 Oral candidiasis

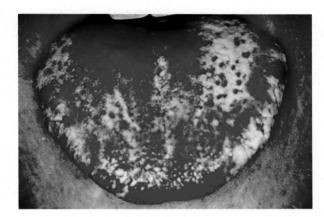

Local Examination

- Inspection of the oral cavity should include a thorough dental evaluation. Edentulousness (Fig. 3.3) alone constitutes oral dysphagia and risks boluses being too large or coarse for proper passage through the pharynx. Poorly fitting dentures or a missing denture could suggest foreign body aspiration leading to obstruction. Other oral pathologies associated with oral dysphagia include mucositis (aphthous ulcers, herpes, etc.) (Fig. 3.4), reduced salivation (Sjögren syndrome, antihistamines, anticholinergic drugs, etc.), or intraoral tumors (Fig. 3.5).
- Indirect laryngoscopy: it was the mainstay of diagnosis of oropharyngeal dysphagia until the advent of video laryngoscopy. One can identify tongue base lesions, ulcers, and tumors of the epiglottis, vallecula, posterior or lateral pharyngeal wall, or foreign bodies like fish bones embedded in the lingual tonsils or inflammation of the arytenoids and vocal cord palsy. The true vocal folds may not approximate completely due to paralysis or arytenoid dislocation or tumor

Fig. 3.5 Tumor left tonsil
(*arrow*)

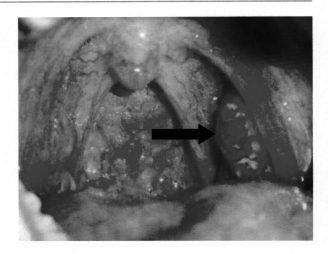

leading to diminished airway protection. This can result in aspiration and dysphagia.

- Evaluating patients with tracheostomy: In these patients, swallowing evaluation can be performed after deflating the pressure cuff and occluding the cannula. This restores trans-glottic airflow and facilitates speech and cough reflex. However occluding the cannula may not be possible in patients with a long–standing tracheostomy or in those with a permanent tracheostoma. Presence of secretions above the cuff, seen after deflating the cuff indicates laryngeal incompetence.
- *Bed side swallow test*: it can be done by administering small pieces of ice along with 3–4 ml of water and semisolids, e.g., purée. The patient's chewing efficacy, movements of the tongue, mandible, floor of the mouth, and larynx are observed as well as palpated. Auscultation of the neck before, during, and after a swallow helps to determine whether there are any secretions or liquids in the pharynx or larynx.
- *FEES:* (Figs. 3.6 and 3.7) Flexible nasopharyngolaryngoscopy is currently the main method of assessing swallowing disorders. Being a dynamic technique, one can visualize all the phases of swallowing, while they occur along with the anatomical appearance of the oropharynx, larynx, and the laryngopharynx. It is a useful tool for diagnosis as well as reassessment of dysphagia disorder.

Other Investigations

- *Videofluoroscopy*: it is currently the gold standard for the study of oropharyngeal dysphagia [9]. Using a flexible nasopharyngolaryngoscope, one can visualize all the phases of swallowing as they occur. It can be used to precisely measure oropharyngeal transit times and diagnose laryngeal penetration (i.e., the foreign material is retained within the laryngeal vestibular zone, extending no further than the true vocal cords) or bronchial aspiration (the foreign material extends beyond the true vocal cords) [9, 10].

Fig. 3.6 Laryngoscopy
showing post-cricoid pooling
(*arrow*)

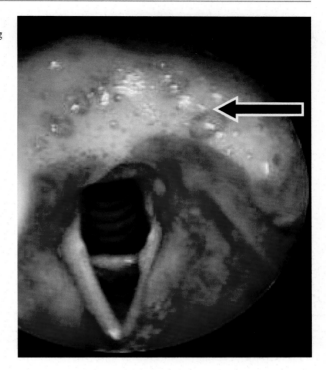

Fig. 3.7 Laryngoscopy
showing edema of right
arytenoid (*arrow*) secondary
to tumor

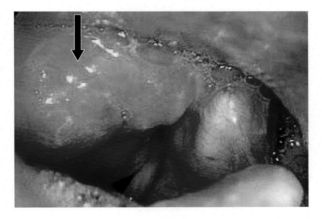

- Evan's methylene blue test: it is useful to diagnose dysphagia and aspiration in tracheostomized patients. It can be performed in those tracheostomized patients who can tolerate cuff deflation and are able to either breathe spontaneously or are able to maintain continuous positive pressure ventilation. A few drops of methylene blue are instilled on the tongue in the semi-sitting position. Appearance of blue-stained secretions in the tracheal aspirations over the next few hours is an indication of aspiration, i.e., a passage from the pharynx to the trachea.

The anatomical level at which normal airway defense reflexes are present can be identified from the timing of the cough with the appearance of methylene blue in the tracheostomy cannula:

Laryngeal during the first 30s, tracheal between 30s and 2 min, and bronchial when longer than 2 min [11].

- *Esophagogastroscopy, manometry,* and other radiological tests: these are discussed in subsequent chapters.

Classification of Dysphagia According to the Degree of Functional Impairment

This classification is typically used in patients with neurological, muscular, or neuromuscular disorders [12].

- *Mild dysphagia* is predominantly oral dysphagia. It is characterized by a delay in swallowing, with loss of oral content, and difficulty in forming the food bolus. There is no dysphonia or cough observed after swallowing in these patients, and there is a very low risk of either airway penetration or aspiration.
- *Moderate dysphagia* is characterized by a predominance of oral and pharyngeal dysfunction. There is a loss of oral content due to lip incontinence and food leakage through the nasal passages. In addition, the transport of the food bolus transport is slowed due to altered lip and tongue contractility. It may be associated with dysphonia, and there may be a risk of laryngeal penetration and/or bronchial aspiration.
- *Severe dysphagia*: In severe dysphagia, there is alteration of the oral and pharyngeal phases of swallowing, along with laryngeal impairment and alteration of the protective airway reflexes. Food remnants are often retained in the pharyngeal recesses, and patients may experience alteration or abolition of laryngeal and hyoid elevation and anteversion during swallowing. Coughing is not always observed.

These individuals are at a high risk of airway penetration and/or aspiration.

Conclusion

Etiology of dysphagia can often be discerned from history and examination of the patient. Therefore, a detailed history eliciting onset, duration, and associated complaints can enable a different tests.

Case 1

A 50-year-old obese man complains of progressively increasing dysphagia to solids. He has a 10-year history of heartburn. He was advised lifestyle modifications and has been treated with proton pump inhibitors. What is the preliminary diagnosis?

Answer: Peptic (Schatzki) rings. It is a ring due to narrowing of the mucosal tissue lining the esophagus [13]. Symptomatic rings may require endoscopy with dilatation.

Case 2

A 45-year-old woman complains of dysphagia and weight loss. Her upper gastrointestinal endoscopy is normal. Barium swallow shows tubular esophagus with a tight lower esophageal sphincter. What is the next test to confirm the diagnosis?

Answer: Esophageal manometry. The patient probably has achalasia with increased tone of the lower esophageal sphincter. This can be confirmed with manometry.

Case 3

A 30-year-old young man is woken up every night with wheezing. He has no history of hypertension, asthma, or snoring. What tests are required to confirm the diagnosis?

Answer: FEES followed by 24 h ambulatory pH studies.

Case 4

A 27-year-old woman with long-standing history of "food getting stuck in her throat" comes for weakness, weight loss, and progressively worsening dysphagia. What tests will she require to confirm the diagnosis?

Answer: An indirect laryngoscopy may show either pooling of saliva in the post-cricoid region and pyriform fossa or a post-cricoid mass. Flexible laryngoscopy with suctioning of the pooled secretions will enable a better visualization of the underlying pathology. If no pathology is seen, then the patient will require an upper esophagoscopy to look for a post-cricoid mass.

Case 5

A 55-year-old man complains of dysphagia, cough, and foul smell emanating from his mouth. He occasionally has regurgitation of undigested food particles. What is the probable diagnosis?

Answer: Pharyngoesophageal diverticulum. Barium swallow and upper gastro-esophagoscopy will confirm the diagnosis.

Case 6

A 65-year-old postmenopausal woman with long-standing history of diabetes complains of dysphagia. She is on antidiabetics and medications for osteoporosis. What is the probable diagnosis?

Answer: She probably has medication associated (pill) esophagitis. Alendronates (for osteoporosis) along with gastroparesis due to long-standing diabetes could have precipitated the condition. She should be advised to sit upright for at least 90 min after intake of medication. If her symptoms persist, she may require an endoscopy and dilatation of a stricture, if present.

References

1. Lee GS, et al. Intermittent dysphagia for solids associated with a multi-ringed esophagus: clinical features and response to dilatation. Dysphagia. 2007;22:55–62.
2. Johnsson F, et al. Symptoms and endoscopic findings in the diagnosis of gastroesophageal reflux disease. Scand J Gastroentol. 1987;22:714–8.
3. Edwards D. Discriminatory value of symptoms in the differential diagnosis of dysphagia. Clin Gastroenterol. 1976;5:49–57.
4. Howard P, et al. Five year prospective study of the incidence, clinical features, and diagnosis of achalasia in Edinburgh. Gut. 1992;33:1011–5.
5. Rosenzweig S, Traube M. The diagnosis and misdiagnosis of achalasia. A study of 25 consecutive patients. J Clin Gastroenterol. 1989;11:147–53.
6. Eckardt VF, et al. Chest pain in achalasia: patient characteristics and clinical course. Gastroenterology. 1999;116:1300–4.
7. Aviv JE, Martin JH, Jones ME, Wee TA, Diamond B, Keen MS, Blitzer A. Age related changes in pharyngeal and supraglottic sensation. Ann Otol Rhinol Laryngol. 1994;103:749–52.
8. Sonies BC. Oropharyngeal dysphagia in the elderly. Clin Geriatr Med. 1992;8(3):569–77.
9. Dodds WJ, Stewart ET, Logemann JA. Physiology and radiology of the normal oral and pharyngeal phases of swallowing. AJR Am J Roentgenol. 1990;154:953–63.
10. Stoeckli SJ, Huisman TA, Seifert B, Martin-Harris BJ. Interrater reliability of videofluoroscopic swallow evaluation. Dysphagia. 2003;18:53–7.
11. Cameron JL, Reynolds J, Zuidema GD. Aspiration in patients with tracheostomies. Surg Gynecol Obstet. 1973;136:68–70.
12. Zambrana-Toledo González N. El mantenimiento de las orientaciones logopédicas en el paciente con disfagia orofaríngea de origen neurogénico. Rev Neurol. 2001;32:986–9.
13. Schatzki R, Gary JE. Dysphagia due to a diaphragm-like localized narrowing in the lower esophagus (lower esophageal ring). Am J Roentgenol Radium Ther Nucl Med. 1953;70(6):911–22. PMID 13104726.

Assessment of Swallowing Disorders

4

Rita Patel

Introduction

Difficulty with swallowing, also known as dysphagia, is a common condition. The prevalence of dysphagia ranges from 16 to 22 % [1, 2]. Dysphagia in adults could be due to a number of causes, primarily including neurological causes, aging, and head and neck cancer. Over the past decade, the assessment of dysphagia has been continually evolving, with speech-language pathologist services being increasingly sought after for the management of individuals with dysphagia. Assessment of dysphagia is multidisciplinary. The members of a multidisciplinary team vary depending on the primary causes of dysphagia. However, the core team members involved in the assessment of dysphagia often include a speech-language pathologist, otolaryngologist, radiologist, gastroenterologist, and dietician. Accurate assessment of individuals with dysphagia is critical to decrease morbidity secondary to aspiration pneumonia and reduce the health-care costs associated with long-term hospitalization for management of aspiration pneumonia [3].

Comprehensive assessment of dysphagia involves a clinical dysphagia assessment and instrumental assessment. Recently, several patient self-assessment scales have been reported that quantify the impact of dysphagia on the quality of life. This chapter focuses on evaluation of adults with dysphagia within the purview of the speech-language pathologist.

R. Patel, PhD, CCC-SLP
Department of Speech and Hearing Sciences,
Indiana University, 200 S. Jordan Avenue, C145,
Bloomington, IN 47405-7002, USA
e-mail: patelrir@indiana.edu

© Springer India 2015
G. Mankekar (ed.), *Swallowing – Physiology, Disorders, Diagnosis and Therapy*,
DOI 10.1007/978-81-322-2419-8_4

Clinical Dysphagia Assessment

The clinical evaluation of swallowing function is the first critical level of assessment for determining the nature of dysphagia. It is defined as an "organized goal-directed evaluation of a variety of interrelated and integrated components of the swallowing process" [4] (p. 13). A comprehensive clinical assessment of swallow function should enable the clinician to describe the nature of the patient's problem, make preliminary determination of a potential diagnosis or cause of the swallowing dysfunction, make judgments regarding aspiration, and make a decision regarding the need for instrumental assessment. The clinical dysphagia assessment consists of a comprehensive case history, examination of the structure and function of the oral mechanism, and trial swallows.

Case History

Comprehensive case history is the first level of assessment for obtaining current and past medical and feeding history. In an outpatient setup, the comprehensive case history can be obtained from the patient, the family members, and/or the caregivers, whereas in an inpatient setup, a comprehensive case history can be obtained from chart review and discussions with the treating team members, in addition to the patient, the family members, and/or the caregivers if possible.

A detailed history should account for the patient's chief complaint; onset of the condition; progression of the condition since the onset; type of the dysphagia (solids, liquids, pills); duration of meal times, recent pneumonia; weight loss; increased body temperature; recent hospitalizations; present and past medical/surgical history; social history/habits regarding hydration; caffeine intake; smoking; and associated symptoms (voice change, shortness of breath, coughing). Patients who are aware of the disorder are often highly accurate in the description and identification of the swallowing problem.

Oral Mechanism Examination

Based on the patient's chief complaint and the clinician's intuition of the patient's problem from the case history, specific components for examination of the oral mechanism can be expanded. Most traditional examination of the oral mechanism involves evaluation of the structure, range of motion, strength, endurance, and sensation of the lips, tongue, palate, mandible, dentition, and larynx. During observation of the structure and function of the oral mechanism, judgments are made regarding the integrity of the cranial nerves that are important in swallowing. Additionally, it is critical to observe the nature of the patient's volitional swallow, which provides insights into the coordination among the various structures and the patient's ability to handle secretions. Pocketing of secretions and/or food on one side indicates a sensory and/or motor involvement on the involved side. Patient's oral hygiene also provides useful indicators of the patient's motor and sensory involvement as well as the patient's cognitive status.

Trial Swallows

The selection of the best food/liquid consistency for trial swallows depends on the information obtained from the case history and oral mechanism examination. It is best to begin trial swallows with a consistency that the patient does not have difficulty with. Often it may be safe to start with a nectar-thick consistency and subsequently increase/decrease the viscosity of the material presented based on the information gathered from the case history. In individuals with severe reduction in the range of motion of the oral structures, it may be best to begin the trial swallows by presenting ice chips, as these can be easily suctioned if needed. Often it is recommended to start with a 5-ml bolus presented via a teaspoon [5]. Depending on the results from the initial bolus presentation, the size of the bolus can be increased. Further one can assess the safety of the bolus when presented via cup and straw.

During the trial swallows, judgments regarding involvement of the base of the tongue, timing of the swallow, and the hyolaryngeal excursion can be made by placing the fingers under the chin; with the index finger positioned behind the mandible, the middle finger on the hyoid bone, the third finger on the thyroid notch, and the fourth finger at the bottom of the thyroid cartilage [5]. After swallowing the bolus, the patients are asked to immediately phonate/a/for approximately 3 s to determine any changes in the voice quality. Gurgling and wet voice quality, in addition to an immediate or delayed cough, could be signs indicative of aspiration. Sensitivity and specificity of the clinical assessment of dysphagia can be increased by using pulse oximetry. Lim et al. [6] reported that combining the pulse oximetry with trial swallows of 50 ml of water during the clinical dysphagia assessment, the sensitivity for detecting aspiration was 100 % and the specificity was 71 % in individuals with acute stroke.

The clinical dysphagia assessment also often known as "bedside" assessment, though invaluable is able to only provide rudimentary information regarding the oropharyngeal stage of swallowing and of frank aspiration. Detailed physiology of the pharyngeal phase in terms of bolus transit time, entry of bolus into the airway, and coordination of the pharyngeal and laryngeal structures during swallow is unavailable from the clinical dysphagia assessment. Physiology of the esophageal phase of swallow also cannot be discerned from the clinical dysphagia assessment.

Instrumental Assessments of Dysphagia

Silent aspiration occurs in approximately 40 % of the individuals presenting with the complaint of dysphagia at bedside [5]. Hence, it is critical to perform instrumental assessment of swallow in individuals that are suspected or at high risk of developing dysphagia. Instrumental assessment of dysphagia also provides useful information regarding the biomechanics and physiology of the impaired mechanism that is useful for determining appropriate management strategies. According to the American Speech-Language Hearing Associations Clinical Practice Guidelines on "clinical indicators for instrumental assessment of dysphagia" [7], instrumental assessment of dysphagia is indicated for effective management of individuals suspected or at risk of swallowing disorders, based on clinical swallow evaluation, when: "(1) the patient's signs and symptoms are inconsistent with findings on the clinical examination, (2) there is a need to confirm a suspected medical diagnosis and/or assist in the determination of a differential diagnosis, (3) confirmation and/or differential diagnosis of the dysphagia is needed, (4) there is either nutritional or pulmonary compromise and a question of whether the oropharyngeal dysphagia is contributing to these conditions, (5) the safety and efficiency of the swallow remains a concern, (6) the patient is identified as a swallow rehabilitation candidate and specific information is needed to guide management and treatment. An instrumental examination is not indicated when: (1) the patient is too medically unstable to tolerate a procedure, (2) the patient is unable to cooperate or participate in an instrumental examination, and (3) in the speech-language pathologist's judgment, the instrumental examination would not change the clinical management of the patient."

Two of the most commonly used instrumental assessments of swallowing include modified barium swallow study and fiberoptic endoscopic examination of swallow. More recently, newer instrumental assessments like flexible fiberoptic examination of swallow function with sensory testing and manometry are beginning to come within the scope of the speech-language pathologists. The choice of the instrumental assessment procedure depends on the evaluation of the signs and the symptoms on clinical evaluation of swallowing. The overall goal of the instrumental assessment is to establish the presence or absence of dysphagia; delineate the resulting physiological disturbances within the oral, pharyngeal, and/or the esophageal phases causing the dysphagia; determine a diet of thin and solid consistencies that is the least restrictive and safe for the patient to maintain adequate nutrition; and determine appropriate treatment plan.

Modified Barium Swallow Study

Modified barium swallow (MBS) is a videofluoroscopic examination of swallow function that provides real-time information of the bolus flow through the oral, pharyngeal, and esophageal phases of swallow. In addition to the information of the different phases of swallowing, MBS provides real-time information regarding the coordination between the phases of swallowing and information regarding the swallow physiology during and after swallow.

The MBS is a multidisciplinary examination of swallow function involving partnership between the speech-language pathologist and the radiologist. The test requires a videofluoroscopic unit with capability of recording the video, appropriate chair for positioning the patient to obtain a good lateral view of the structures

Fig. 4.1 Lateral view on modified barium swallow study of a patient with a tracheostomy tube and a nasogastric tube. This example shows stasis in the vallecular with shallow penetration into the pyriform sinus post swallow

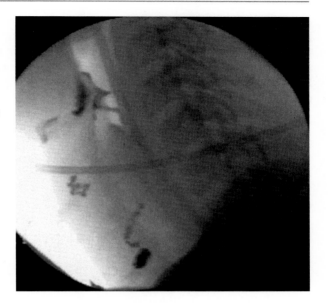

involved in swallowing, different grades of barium bolus consistencies of known viscosity (e.g., thin liquids, nectar-thick liquids, honey thick liquids, solids, and barium pill), and foods that the patient has expressed difficulty swallowing. A universally excepted protocol for MBS does not exist. The MBS usually starts with the consistency that the patient will have least difficulty with (e.g., nectar-thick liquids or thin liquids). Depending on the results with the initial consistency, consistencies of honey thick, pudding, solids, and pills are presented. It is generally safe to present small portions initially (e.g., teaspoon). If the patient is successful with the teaspoon amount for a specific consistency, subsequent presentations should test rapid sequential intake of the consistency that mimics bolus intake during meal times. If penetration and/or aspiration are observed, it is critical to perform appropriate compensatory strategies or swallow maneuvers (e.g., chin tuck, left/right head turn, Mendelsohn maneuver) to determine their success in preventing penetration and/or aspiration.

Examination of the swallowing function on MBS is initially performed using a lateral view (Fig. 4.1). After the examination in the lateral view, the clinician typically proceeds with the examination using the frontal view. The frontal view provides information regarding the symmetry between the left and right side of the pharyngeal structures. Information regarding the proximal part of the esophagus can also be obtained using the frontal view. Often during this view, the entire esophagus could be scanned to examine for distal and proximal portions of the esophagus and intraesophageal reflux.

The MBS studies are often visually rated by the speech pathologist to determine the bolus transit time through the various phases of swallowing, location and cause of the stasis, compensatory maneuvers useful for partially or completely eliminating the stasis, timing of the swallow reflex, coordination of the structures involved in the swallow reflex, amount of aspiration/penetration, causes of aspiration/penetration, and compensatory strategies responsible for eliminating the penetration/aspiration. The eight-step penetration and aspiration scale developed by Rosenbek et al. [8] can be used to evaluate the degree of penetration and aspiration observed on MBS. The eight steps are:

1. Material does not enter airway
2. Remains above folds/ejected from airway
3. Remains above folds/not ejected from airway
4. Contacts folds/ejected from airway
5. Contacts folds/not ejected from airway
6. Passes below folds/ejected into larynx or out of airway
7. Passes below folds/not ejected despite effort
8. Passes below folds/no spontaneous effort to eject

In order to compare findings across clinics, it is critical to establish a minimum standard clinical protocol for evaluation and interpretation of findings that can be used across clinics. Martin-Harris et al. [9] reported a protocol called the new Modified Barium Swallowing Study Tool (MBSImP™©) that standardized the administration of contrast viscosities and reporting methods for the MBS. The MBSImP™© was tested in a heterogeneous sample of 300 patients to observed 17 well-defined physiologic swallowing components of lip closure, hold position/tongue control, bolus preparation/mastication, bolus transport/lingual motion, oral residue, initiation of the pharyngeal swallow, soft palate elevation, laryngeal elevation, anterior hyoid motion, epiglottic movement, laryngeal closure, pharyngeal stripping wave, pharyngeal contraction, PES opening, tongue base retraction, pharyngeal residue, and esophageal clearance in the upright position. Evaluation of the standardized MBSImP™© revealed high inter- and intra-rate reliability. Though MBSImP™© is useful, evaluation of the MBS relies on making visual perceptual judgments, which may be hard to compare across clinics.

Kendall et al. [10] reported a paradigm involving quantitative evaluation of the of MBS studies known as dynamic swallow study (DSS). The DSS allows objective evaluation of 17 measures that can be plotted for liquid boluses of 1, 3, and 20 cc. The 17 measures represent displacement and timing measurements, e.g., bolus transit, pharyngeal transit, oropharyngeal transit and hypopharyngeal transit, swallow gestures, soft palate elevation, aryepiglottic fold elevation, hyoid bone elevation, pharyngoesophageal sphincter opening, pharyngeal constriction, and epiglottic return. Objective evaluation of MBS represents an improvement over subjective reporting as it allows for evaluation of the examination without bias and makes it possible to assess subtle changes in swallowing function between and within subjects over time.

MBS is the mainstay for assessment of dysphagia. However, it does result in radiation exposure depending on the length of the study. Some patient's may not be able to tolerate barium or could have an adverse allergic reaction to barium, which

Standard flexible endoscope   **Distal chip-tip flexible endoscope**

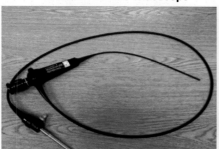 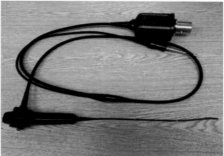

Fig. 4.2 Types of flexible endoscopes that can be used for fiberoptic endoscopic examination of swallow (FEES)

however is rare. Sometimes, because of the cognitive or physical limitation of size, it may not be able to position the patient upright for adequate imaging. In such instances, alternatives to MBS are often used for instrumental assessment of swallowing function.

Fiberoptic Endoscopic Examination of Swallow

Fiberoptic endoscopic examination of swallow (FEES) involves the use of a transnasal fiberoptic endoscope for evaluation of swallowing function. FEES was first introduced by Langmore et al. in 1988 [11] and has gained widespread popularity since its initial introduction. A standard fiberoptic or a distal chip tip endoscope can be introduced through the nasal passage unilaterally to visualize certain events of the oral transfer phase and the pharyngeal phase of swallow (Fig. 4.2). During FEES, it is recommended to place the tip of the endoscope in the pharyngeal area around the midportion of the base of the tongue rather than the laryngeal area to enable visualization of the bolus transit. Clinicians vary regarding their use of topical anesthetic to the nasal mucosa for examination of the swallow function. Topical anesthetic when used is used minimally to prevent any adverse effects of topical anesthetic on the pharyngeal mucosa.

Premature spillage of bolus into the vallecula; base of tongue retraction; penetration of the bolus into the laryngeal vestibule (Fig. 4.3); stasis in the pyriform and vallecular spaces (Fig. 4.4) are some of the physiologic events that can be observed using FEES. In addition to the swallow physiology, FEES enables the clinician for evaluation of laryngeal structures and edema/erythema of the laryngeal structures due to laryngopharyngeal reflux. Typically, boluses of known viscosity are colored with green or blue dye for ease of visualization of possible penetration or aspiration on FEES. Compensatory maneuvers can be used during the test to ascertain their effectiveness in improving the safety of swallowing. FEES is particular beneficial for examining the structures of the larynx, location and severity of the stasis, and in

Fig. 4.3 Fiberoptic
endoscopic examination of
swallow (FEES) revealing
premature spillage of liquid
into the laryngeal vestibule

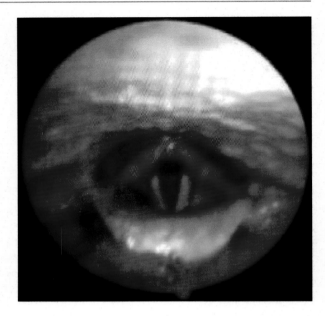

Fig. 4.4 Fiberoptic
endoscopic examination of
swallow (FEES) revealing
stasis in the vallecular space

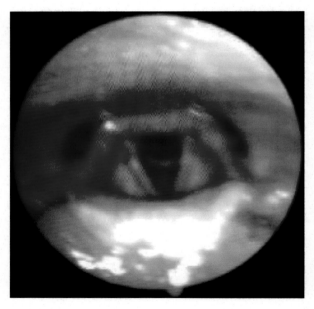

providing biofeedback for the correct use of compensatory maneuvers or training
exercises to improve swallow function. Some examples of compensatory strategies
that can be used with FEES include modification of the bolus consistency and volume, changing the rate of delivery of the bolus, and modification of the sequence of
bolus delivery. Some examples of therapeutic strategies that can be evaluated with

FEES include effortful swallow, breath hold maneuver, base of tongue exercises, and thermal-tactile stimulation. FEES is particularly advantageous for evaluating of swallow function in critically ill patients at bedside and in determining the patient readiness for swallowing postradiation or robotic surgery for treatment of oropharyngeal carcinoma.

Flexible endoscopic evaluation of swallow with sensory testing (FEEST) is a modality where both sensory and motor tests for swallowing can be performed, unlike FEES, which only examines the motor component of swallowing. FEEST was first introduced by Aviv et al. in 1993 [12]. FEEST examines the laryngeal closure reflex, which is critical for the airway protection. Pressure and duration of calibrated pulses of air are delivered to the hypopharyngeal tissue, which is known to be innervated by the superior laryngeal nerve that triggers the laryngeal adductor reflex [13]. Several studies have been conducted demonstrating a positive relationship between edema of the hypopharyngeal structures and reduction in the laryngeal airway reflex on FEEST examination [14, 15]. Specialized equipment that delivers calibrated puffs of air is required for FEEST and has not received widespread usage across clinics.

FEES and FEEST are unable to provide all the information necessary across the different phases of swallowing. Information regarding bolus management in the oral phase of the swallowing is not available from FEES and FEEST. Another limitation of FEES and FEEST is that during the moment of swallow, there is "white out" from contraction of the pharyngeal wall against the tip of the endoscope, and hence information regarding the degree of pharyngeal contraction, upper esophageal opening, and hyolaryngeal excursion cannot be obtained from these examinations. Similarly, it is difficult to visualize penetration and aspiration during the swallow. However, despite of the above limitations, recent studies have reported that FEES provides comparable information compared to the MBS regarding the overall diagnosis of dysphagia and treatment strategies for safe swallow [16].

Manometry

Manometry is an instrumental assessment procedure that provides detailed information regarding the peristaltic pressure waves involved in the process of swallowing. Frequently for esophageal manometry three tubes are placed, one at the site of the upper esophageal segment, the second within the esophagus, and the third at the lower esophageal segment [5]. Esophageal manometry is helpful for identification of the motility disorders affecting the esophagus, particularly aperistalsis and failure of the lower esophageal sphincter to relax [17].

More recently pharyngeal manometry is an investigation that has been identified as being part of the emerging area of practice for the speech-language pathologist [18]. Pharyngeal manometry can be performed in conjunction with esophageal manometry or in isolation. Data from pharyngeal manometry can be examined both qualitatively as well as quantitatively. A polyvinyl tube made up of multiple pressure sensors is passed transnasally and the patient is instructed to perform a series of dry swallows. With advances in technology, high-resolution pharyngeal manometry has provided a complete picture of the pharyngeal pressure patterns [18]. It is simpler to perform and provides the clinician with an image that is easily interpretable compared to traditional manometry. Saline boluses of various sizes are used for high-resolution manometry. Estimates of pressures (mmHg) at various locations within the pharynx can be obtained. Pharyngeal manometry can be particularly useful for differentiating between muscular weakness versus stricture of the upper esophageal segment. There is emerging evidence that the pharyngeal manometry can also be used to measure treatment outcomes in individuals with dysphagia [18].

Patient Self-Assessment Tools

The patient self-assessment tools provide useful information regarding the degree of the swallowing impairment on the patient's quality of life. Two widely used scales for estimating the impact of the swallowing dysfunction on the quality of life include the MD Anderson Dysphagia Inventory and the SWAL-QOL.

The MD Anderson Dysphagia Inventory (MDADI) is a 20-item scale that involves assessment of four domains of global, emotional, function, and physical subscales of patient's response to swallowing the quality of life following head and neck cancer treatment [19]. The MDADI was validated on 100 consecutive subjects with neoplasm of the aerodigestive tract and was reported to have high reliability and internal consistency [19]. The scores can range from 0 to 100, with higher values indicative of superior perception of swallowing ability.

The SWAL-QOL tool when initially developed was a 93-item quality-of-life and quality-of-case outcomes tool for dysphagia in patients that are elderly and chronically ill [20]. The SWAL-QOL was reduced from 93 items to a 44-item tool and 15 items in the SWAL-CARE revised version [21]. The SWAL-QOL and the SWAL-CARE differentiate patients with dysphagia from patients with normal swallowing and hence can be used with any patients with dysphagia. The scale was reported to be sensitive to the severity of the oropharyngeal dysphagia and was reported to have high internal consistency and short-term reproducibility [21].

Summary

Dysphagia is swallowing difficulty; the inability of which will significantly influence the overall health and nutrition status of the affected individual and in turn negatively affects their quality of life. Timely and accurate assessment of dysphagia is critical, as failure of which has the potential to lead to fatal consequences. The tools available in the clinical armamentarium of the speech-language pathologist are continually expanding. Comprehensive clinical examination of dysphagia is multidisciplinary the speech-language pathologists playing a pivotal role. To evaluate dysphagia, a thorough case history and clinical evaluation of swallow dysfunction provides key guiding principles for decision making regarding the choice of instrumental procedures. One or more of the instrumental procedures may be needed to obtain detailed understanding regarding the impaired physiology leading to aspiration. Appropriate assessment of dysphagia is a team effort involving multiple disciplines. It is the role of the speech-language pathologists to make appropriate referrals, when indicated for comprehensive assessment of dysphagia. Collaboration among the various professions is critical for optimal management of dysphagia. As the field continues to evolve, standardized objective evaluations would be available to the clinicians that can be compared across clinics.

References

1. Bloem BR, Lagaay AM, van Beek W, Haan J, Roos RA, Wintzen AR. Prevalence of subjective dysphagia in community residents aged over 87. BMJ. 1990;300:721–2.
2. Kjellen G, Tibbling L. Manometric oesophageal function, acid perfusion test and symptomatology in a 55-year-old general population. Clin Physiol. 1981;1:405–15.
3. Odderson IR, Keatron J, McKenna BS. Swallow management in patients on an acute stroke pathway: quality is cost effective. Arch Phys Med Rehabil. 1995;76:1130–3.
4. Langemore SE, Logemann JA. After the clinical bedsider examination: what next? J Speech Lang Pathol. 1991;9:13–20.
5. Logemann JA. Evaluation and treatment of swallowing disorders. San Diego: College-Hill Press; 1983.
6. Lim SH, Lieu PK, Phua SY, et al. Accuracy of bedside clinical methods compared with fiberoptic endoscopic examination of swallowing (FEES) in determining the risk of aspiration in acute stroke patients. Dysphagia. 2001;16:1–6.
7. American Speech-Language-Hearing Association. Clinical indicators for instrumental assessment of dysphagia [Guidelines]. Available from www.asha.org/policy. 2000.
8. Rosenbek JC, Robbins JA, Roecker EB, Coyle JL, Wood JL. A penetration-aspiration scale. Dysphagia. 1996;11:93–8.
9. Martin-Harris B, Brodsky MB, Michel Y, et al. MBS measurement tool for swallow impairment–MBSImp: establishing a standard. Dysphagia. 2008;23:392–405.
10. Kendall KA, McKenzie S, Leonard RJ, Goncalves MI, Walker A. Timing of events in normal swallowing: a videofluoroscopic study. Dysphagia. 2000;15:74–83.
11. Langmore SE, Schatz K, Olsen N. Fiberoptic endoscopic examination of swallowing safety: a new procedure. Dysphagia. 1988;2:216–9.
12. Aviv JE, Martin JH, Keen MS, Debell M, Blitzer A. Air pulse quantification of supraglottic and pharyngeal sensation: a new technique. Ann Otol Rhinol Laryngol. 1993;102:777–80.
13. Bastian RW, Riggs LC. Role of sensation in swallowing function. Laryngoscope. 1999;109:1974–7.
14. Aviv JE. Prospective, randomized outcome study of endoscopy versus modified barium swallow in patients with dysphagia. Laryngoscope. 2000;110:563–74.
15. Jafari S, Prince RA, Kim DY, Paydarfar D. Sensory regulation of swallowing and airway protection: a role for the internal superior laryngeal nerve in humans. J Physiol. 2003;550:287–304.
16. Langmore SE, Schatz K, Olson N. Endoscopic and videofluoroscopic evaluations of swallowing and aspiration. Ann Otol Rhinol Laryngol. 1991;100:678–81.
17. Spechler SJ, Castell DO. Classification of oesophageal motility abnormalities. Gut. 2001;49:145–51.
18. Knigge MA, Thibeault S, McCulloch TM. Implementation of high-resolution manometry in the clinical practice of speech language pathology. Dysphagia. 2014;29:2–16.

19. Chen AY, Frankowski R, Bishop-Leone J, et al. The development and validation of a dysphagia-specific quality-of-life questionnaire for patients with head and neck cancer: the M. D. Anderson dysphagia inventory. Arch Otolaryngol Head Neck Surg. 2001;127:870–6.
20. McHorney CA, Bricker DE, Robbins J, Kramer AE, Rosenbek JC, Chignell KA. The SWAL-QOL outcomes tool for oropharyngeal dysphagia in adults: II. Item reduction and preliminary scaling. Dysphagia. 2000;15:122–33.
21. McHorney CA, Robbins J, Lomax K, et al. The SWAL-QOL and SWAL-CARE outcomes tool for oropharyngeal dysphagia in adults: III. Documentation of reliability and validity. Dysphagia. 2002;17:97–114.

Endoscopic Diagnosis and Management of Swallowing Disorders

5

Rajesh Sainani and Deepak Gupta

Approach to Dysphagia

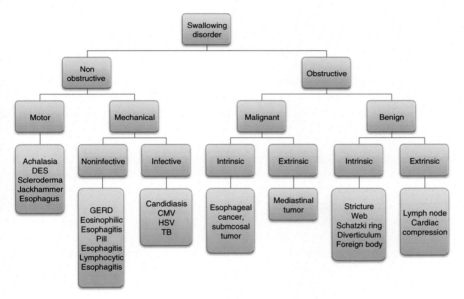

R. Sainani, MD, DNB [Gastro] (✉)
Department of Gastroenterology, Jaslok Hospital, Mumbai, India
e-mail: drsainani@gmail.com

D. Gupta, MD, DNB [Gastro]
Department of Gastroenterology, KEM Hospital, Mumbai, India

© Springer India 2015
G. Mankekar (ed.), *Swallowing – Physiology, Disorders, Diagnosis and Therapy*,
DOI 10.1007/978-81-322-2419-8_5

Approach to Esophageal Swallowing Disorder

Dysphagia, odynophagia, retrosternal chest pain, regurgitation, and heartburn are the major symptoms of esophageal disorders. In oropharyngeal dysphagia, there is inability to initiate swallow, nasopharyngeal regurgitation, coughing or choking on attempted eating, or aspiration. Esophageal disorders can be classified as obstructive and nonobstructive etiology. Esophageal diameter less than 15 mm will lead to obstructive disorder and present with dysphagia to solids more in comparison to liquids. Nonobstructive disorders especially motor disorder present with dysphagia to both solids and liquids. Odynophagia, food impaction, or chest pain can also be seen. Dysphagia can be acute as in case of food impaction, pill, and infective esophagitis. Intermittent dysphagia is seen in rings and webs, while progressive dysphagia is seen in malignancy and strictures.

Zenker's Diverticulum

Zenker's diverticulum is a pulsion diverticulum in the hypopharynx. It is an outpouching of the mucosa due to a muscular weakness between cricopharyngeus and inferior pharyngeal constrictor.

There are various hypotheses which may be responsible for developing a Zenker's diverticulum, upper esophageal sphincter [UES] dysfunction-incomplete relaxation, motility disorders of the esophagus, or gastroesophageal reflux disease causing esophageal or UES dysmotility.

This diagnosis is suspected on the history and confirmed on barium examination and upper gastrointestinal endoscopy. The barium shows features of pouch which retains the barium. The neck of the pouch is above the cricopharyngeal sphincter. On upper gastrointestinal endoscopy, the diverticulum can be visualized. The presence of carcinoma in situ or squamous cell carcinoma needs to be excluded. One must be careful and push the endoscope blindly to prevent perforation of the diverticulum.

Esophageal manometry is not required in all cases, but it may help underline an existing esophageal motility disorder like esophageal spasm or achalasia cardia or ineffective esophageal motility.

Flexible endoscopic treatment of diverticulum involves dividing the bridge between the diverticulum and the esophagus. This can be done by argon plasma coagulation, needle knife, or a monopolar forceps. The use of Zenker's diverticuloscope or the hood or the cap over the endoscope has improved the view of the septum during the procedure and protection of the wall. A nasogastric tube in the esophagus provides better exposure of the septum and protects the anterior esophageal wall. The needle knife is used to cut from the septum from the midline towards the inferior part of the diverticulum. The direction of the cut can be from inside the diverticulum towards the posterior esophageal wall or the reverse direction. If one extends beyond the inferior part, perforation occurs. Endoclips may be applied for bleeding or to prevent micro perforation.

Argon plasma coagulation uses a noncontact method to divide the septum. The septum can be divided from below upwards or from above downwards.

Esophageal Diverticulum

Diverticula are outpouchings of one or more layers of the intestinal wall that may occur at any level of the esophagus. Diverticula are classified as true, false, and intramural types depending on the number of intestinal wall layers involved. True diverticula contain all layers of the intestinal wall, false diverticula contain only mucosal and submucosal layers, and intramural diverticula refer to outpouchings contained within the submucosa layer. Diverticula of the body of the esophagus are divided into midthoracic (parabronchial) and epiphrenic diverticula. Diverticula are also classified based on the pathogenesis as pulsion or traction diverticulum. Pulsion diverticulum is due to the high intraluminal pressure against weakness in gastrointestinal tract wall. Traction diverticulum is due to pulling forces on the outside of the esophagus from adjacent inflammatory process (mediastinal lymph node). In the lower esophagus, epiphrenic diverticula are typically considered to be pulsion diverticula. Epiphrenic diverticula are often associated with achalasia.

Mid-esophageal diverticulum may be associated with diffuse esophageal spasm or mediastinal fibrosis. Diffuse intramural diverticulosis or intramural pseudodiverticulosis is a rare entity of multiple 1- to 3-mm mucosal outpouchings associated with inflammation and esophageal wall thickening. It is due to dilation of the esophageal glands.

Midthoracic and epiphrenic diverticula are usually asymptomatic and are discovered during routine radiologic evaluations for unrelated complaints. They mostly occur in middle-aged adults and elderly. Symptoms of dysphagia and regurgitation can be reported by patients, particularly those with diverticula related to diffuse esophageal spasm or achalasia.

On barium swallow, midthoracic or traction diverticulum is typically a small, widemouth pouch located near the tracheal bifurcation. An epiphrenic diverticulum, on the other hand, appears as a large globular pouch, often associated with abnormal esophageal contractions. Endoscopy will help in visualizing the outpouching in the esophagus.

Midthoracic or epiphrenic diverticula that are asymptomatic need not be treated. In symptomatic patients, treatment should be aimed at the underlying esophageal motility disorder or stricture. Surgical management of midthoracic or epiphrenic diverticula depends on the underlying motility disorder which can involve extended myotomy with a diverticulectomy.

Achalasia Cardia

It is defined as a primary motility disorder of the esophagus, in which there is a loss of esophageal peristalsis and insufficient lower esophageal sphincter relaxation.

Achalasia has an equal incidence in men and women and can affect all age groups but is more commonly seen in the third to sixth decade of life. The exact etiology may be autoimmune, viral, or neurodegenerative in nature. In areas where *Trypanosoma cruzi* is endemic, achalasia presents as a manifestation of Chagas disease.

The ganglion cells of the myenteric plexus are degenerated which causes an imbalance in the inhibitory and excitatory neurons of the lower esophageal sphincter. The end result is unopposed action of the cholinergic activity which leads to insufficient relaxation of the lower esophageal sphincter. The manifestations of achalasia are more due to the incompletely relaxation of the lower esophageal sphincter rather than the aperistaltic esophagus. The aperistaltic esophagus usually causes symptoms when it gets massively dilated to form a sigmoid esophagus. Thus, all the treatment modalities are directed towards the lower esophageal sphincter.

Achalasia should be suspected in all patients who present with dysphagia to solids and liquids and in those patients in whom the regurgitation does not respond to proton pump therapy. The disorder starts insidiously and gradually progressive over weeks and months.

Dysphagia to solids and liquids and regurgitation are common symptoms during presentation. Regurgitation usually gets worse during supine posture, and some patients may self-induce vomiting to relieve the symptoms. Many patients will describe the heartburn to be bland in nature because acid does not mix the retained food in the esophagus. Patients may use liquids to push food down and may change posture by arching their neck or pushing their shoulders backwards to help the food go down into the stomach. At times they may complain of heartburn due to residual food in the esophagus. They also complain of chest pain which is usually substernal. Weight loss commonly occurs in patients with achalasia, but if significant weight loss occurs especially in an elderly patient, then secondary achalasia should be excluded.

Endoscopically, the findings show saliva, liquid, and food in the esophagus. The esophagus appears dilated and roomy (Fig. 5.1). There is no evidence of mechanical obstruction seen. If there is long-standing stasis of food, then erythema and

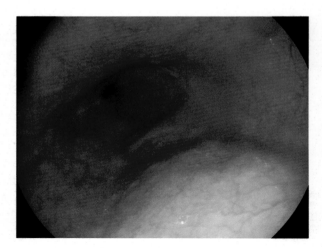

Fig. 5.1 Achalasia cardia dilated esophagus

erosions or candida infection may be seen. There is some resistance in passage of the endoscope from the esophagus into the stomach; a sensation described by endoscopists as a "give way" may be appreciated. This is not mandatory for the diagnosis, but if present in a non-dilated esophagus without residue, it helps the clinician to pursue his/her suspicion of achalasia by asking for a manometry. If there is a massively dilated esophagus like sigmoid esophagus, the lower esophageal sphincter opening may be hidden under the residual food and maybe displaced laterally. Rarely, the endoscopists may find it difficult to intubate the stomach. Endoscopy is recommended in all patients with suspected achalasia to exclude secondary achalasia like a gastroesophageal junction tumor or a fundal tumor infiltrating the gastroesophageal junction.

Manometry is now recommended in all patients before starting therapy. Earlier conventional manometry described achalasia to have aperistaltic esophagus, elevated lower esophageal sphincter resting pressures, and an elevated nadir [residual] pressure of the lower esophageal sphincter of >8 mmHg. Now with the advent of high-resolution manometry, achalasia can be classified into three types by the Chicago classification, which help the clinician decide the therapy that will best benefit the patient.

Type 1 achalasia cardia (Fig. 5.2)
Hundred percent failed peristalsis, mean integrated relaxation pressures [IRP] of the lower esophageal sphincter >15 mmHg

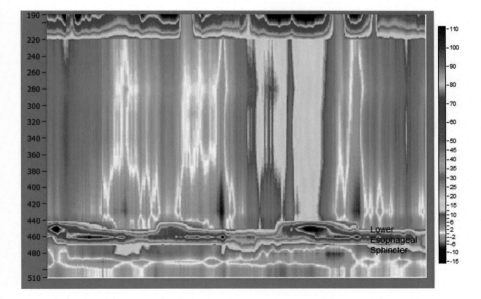

Fig. 5.2 Type 1 achalasia

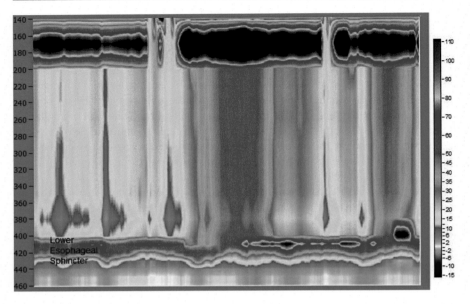

Fig. 5.3 Type 2 achalasia

Type 2 achalasia cardia (Fig. 5.3)
No normal peristalsis, panesophageal pressurization in >20 % of swallows, mean integrated relaxation pressures of the lower esophageal sphincter >15 mmHg

Type 3 achalasia cardia (Fig. 5.4)
No normal peristalsis, preserved fragments of distal peristalsis or premature [spastic] contractions in >20 % of swallows, mean integrated relaxation pressures of the lower esophageal sphincter >15 mmHg

Other Tests

Barium esophagogram will show a dilated esophagus, bird-beak appearance at the lower esophageal sphincter, and holdup of barium above the lower esophageal sphincter with a delay in passage of the barium into the stomach (Fig. 5.5). There will be absent peristalsis in the body of the esophagus. A sigmoid-like esophagus may occur in patients with long-standing untreated disease.

Chest X-ray will usually show a widened mediastinum due to the dilated esophagus and absent gastric air bubble which occurs due to a non-relaxing lower esophageal sphincter.

Treatment

The treatment of achalasia is now influenced by the type of achalasia found on manometry. Type 1 achalasia responds best to laparoscopic Heller's myotomy, and

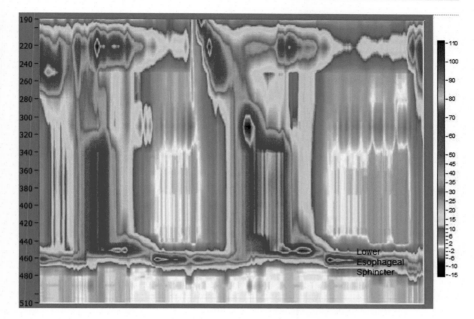

Fig. 5.4 Type 3 achalasia

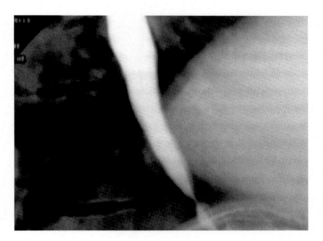

Fig. 5.5 Barium achalasia cardia

type 2 achalasia has equal response rates to laparoscopic Heller's myotomy and pneumatic dilatation, and type 3 does poorly to pneumatic dilatation, botulinum toxin, or laparoscopic Heller's myotomy.

Drug treatment with calcium channel blockers and nitrates has poor response rates up to 10 %. They are usually reserved for patients who are unwell due to comorbidities or refuse treatment. They act by reducing the lower esophageal sphincter pressures.

Botulinum toxin can be injected endoscopically into the lower esophageal sphincter. It acts by blocking the release of acetylcholine from the presynaptic receptors and restores the balance between the inhibitory and excitatory neu-rotransmitters. It is injected in four quadrants, 1 cm above the Z-line of the gas-troesophageal junction in a dose of 25 units [1 ml] in each quadrant. The response is seen in 70–90 % of patients, but most of them would relapse in 6–12 months and will require a second injection. The relapse rate is higher and the time to relapse is earlier when compared to pneumatic dilatation or laparoscopic Heller's myotomy.

Pneumatic dilatation and laparoscopic myotomy are the standard of care for achalasia cardia. The main aim of pneumatic dilation is to disrupt the lower esophageal sphincter. This reduces the gradient across the lower esophageal sphincter and helps the esophagus to empty the food and liquids by gravity. Pneumatic dilatation is done with a Rigiflex dilator after placing a guidewire with the endoscope. Most endoscopists would start with a 30 mm size of the balloon, and if it does not respond, then they would use a high diameter of 35 or 40 mm. The dilator is inflated with air till one can visualize "waist" obliteration of the balloon on fluoroscopy. This balloon is kept inflated for 1 min after which it is rapidly deflated. Some endoscopists would reinflate the balloon once more and note the pressure required for waist obliteration, which will be less than that required the first time. This procedure has a success rate of 70–90 % in expert hands as the initial success, but 50 % of patients would relapse over 5 years. They will then be subjected to another pneumatic dilatation or be sent for laparoscopic Heller's myotomy.

For laparoscopic Heller's myotomy, please refer to the chapter ahead.

Diffuse Esophageal Spasm

This is a motility disorder of the esophagus. The clinical significance of this disor-der is not known. It was also called as distal esophageal spasm because the findings usually occurred in the distal esophagus [smooth muscle]. There is no clarity on the fact if symptoms are produced due to the impaired [rapid] contraction or due to the elevated amplitude that may be observed in some of them.

The common presentation is unexplained chest pain or dysphagia. Gastroesophageal reflux disease [GERD] can also present with the similar symp-toms but usually have heartburn as one of the major symptoms. GERD can be pres-ent in two-thirds of patients with motility disorders, and a 24 h ph study can differentiate primary from secondary esophageal motility disorders. It would be worthwhile doing an endoscopy to exclude any obstructive pathology if dysphagia is a presenting symptom. Cardiac cause for the chest pain should always be excluded before pursuing this diagnosis.

The pathophysiology of diffuse esophageal spasm is not exactly known. But since treatment with nitrates has shown benefit, a defect in the nitric acid synthesis has been postulated.

CT scan may show increase thickness of the esophageal wall to >3 mm in some patients. Since cancer of the esophagus can also present with hypertrophy of the esophageal wall, further investigations to exclude a malignancy are warranted.

The earlier conventional manometry defined diffuse esophageal spasm as:

1. Simultaneous [synchronous] contractions in >20 % of swallows with amplitude >30 mmHg in the distal esophagus
2. Repetitive contractions >3 peaks in the distal esophagus
3. Distal peristaltic velocity >8 cm/s in the distal esophagus

The current Chicago classification for high-resolution manometry classifies diffuse esophageal spasm as:

1. IRP [integrated relaxation pressures] <15 mmHg
   Integrated relaxation pressure [IRP] is measured in mmHg and defined as mean esophageal gastric junction pressure measured for four contiguous or non-contiguous seconds of relaxation in the 10-s window following deglutitive UES relaxation.
2. Distal latency <4.5 s
   Distal latency [DL] is the interval between upper esophageal sphincter relaxation and the contractile deceleration point. The distal latency is >4.5 s in normal peristalsis.
3. Contractile forward velocity >9 cm/s
   Contractile front velocity (cm s−1) [CFV] is the slope of the tangent approximating the 30 mmHg isobaric contour between the proximal trough of the distal esophageal contraction and the contractile deceleration point.

For the management of diffuse esophageal spasm, see below in nutcracker esophagus.

Nutcracker Esophagus

This is a motility disorder of the esophagus in whom there is an elevated amplitude of peristalsis [>180 mmHg] in the distal smooth muscle of the esophagus on conventional manometry (Figs. 5.6 and 5.7).

In the Chicago classification, it is classified as a distal contractile integral >5,000 mmHg-s-cm with an integrated relaxation pressure <15 mmHg.

Distal contractile integral (mmHg-s-cm) [DCI] is defined as amplitude x duration x length of the distal esophageal contraction >20 mmHg from proximal to distal pressure troughs.

The presentation is commonly chest pain, rarely dysphagia since there are no bolus transit abnormalities seen. It may be associated with a hypertensive or hypotensive lower esophageal sphincter. The symptoms usually poorly correlate with the timing of the elevated amplitudes, i.e., not all high-amplitude peristalses cause pain. Visceral hypersensitivity may be responsible in some patients with chest pain.

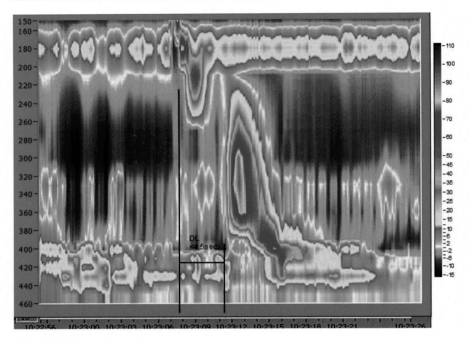

Fig. 5.6 Diffuse esophageal spasm

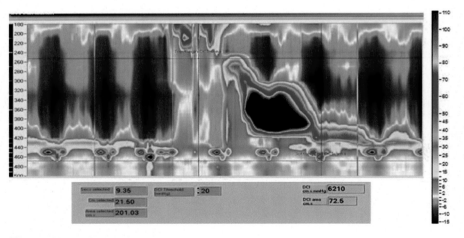

Fig. 5.7 Nutcracker esophagus

Endoscopy in Spastic Disorders of the Esophagus

Endoscopy is usually normal and there are no characteristic signs.

Barium studies may show a corkscrew or rosary bead appearance due to non-propulsive peristalsis.

Management of Diffuse Esophageal Spasm and Nutcracker Esophagus

Drug treatment provides varied degree of relief for spastic disorders of the esophagus.

Reassurance and alleviation of anxiety is important. The fact that a diagnosis has been reached itself is reassuring to many patients. Counseling the patient that it is usually a non-progressive disease and without any long-term adverse outcome helps in alleviation of their anxiety.

Proton Pump Inhibitors
Gastroesophageal reflux disease may also contribute to the chest pain. A trial of proton pump inhibitors in twice daily dosage for 3 months may benefit such patients.

Calcium Channel Blockers
Nifedipine [10–20 mg three times daily] and diltiazem [30–60 mg three to four times daily] both have been used with variable results. They help in alleviating chest pain and dysphagia. Nifedipine can cause pedal edema and diltiazem can cause bradycardia and should not be used with other rate-slowing drugs like beta blockers.

Nitrates
Isosorbide dinitrate can be used before meals in patients with dysphagia or at the time of the chest pain. Headache is a common side effect and tolerance may develop if used for a long duration.

Tricyclic Antidepressants
Imipramine [50 mg/OD] or amitriptyline can be used for chest pain. They help by modifying the visceral hypersensitivity.

Phosphodiesterase Inhibitors
Sildenafil has been shown to help patients with chest pain in nutcracker esophagus. Its action is due to its smooth muscle relaxant effect which can reduce esophageal spastic contractions and the lower esophageal sphincter pressures.

Botulinum Toxin
In patients not responding to drug treatment, botulinum toxin can be used. Its effect is short term [up to 6 months] when injected in the lower esophagus just above the lower esophageal sphincter. Its mechanism of action is by binding to receptors and reducing the amount of acetylcholine release.

Balloon Dilatation
This has been used in diffuse spasm and nutcracker esophagus with partial relief and recurrence of symptoms. Its usual role is in the treatment of achalasia cardia.

Non-pharmacological Treatment

Hot water to be taken with meals has been found to reduce the amplitude of esophageal contraction and improve esophageal clearance.

Peppermint oil has been tried in patients of diffuse esophageal spasm. It was found to improve symptoms of chest pain and improve manometric findings.

Scleroderma

The esophagus is unique by having skeletal muscle in the upper third and smooth muscle in the lower two-third. Scleroderma causes fibrosis and atrophy in the smooth muscle of the esophagus. The disease involves the esophageal body to cause aperistalsis [in the lower two-third of the esophagus] and weakens the lower esophageal sphincter [hypotensive]. The motility of the skeletal muscle [upper third of the esophagus] is unaffected.

Endoscopically, there are no characteristic changes found in the esophagus, but due to a hypotensive lower esophageal sphincter, signs of reflux esophagitis and stricture formation may be seen. The lower esophageal sphincter may appear lax. The esophageal body may be dilated due to aperistalsis of the esophageal body (Fig. 5.8).

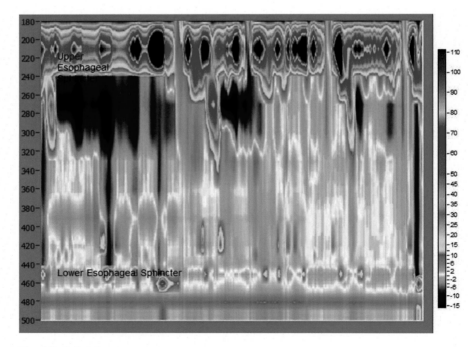

Fig. 5.8 Scleroderma

Manometry shows:

1. Normal peristalsis in the upper third of the esophagus-striated muscle
2. Aperistalsis in the lower two-third of the esophagus-smooth muscle
3. Hypotensive lower esophageal sphincter [<10 mmHg]

Treatment

Proton Pump Inhibitors

Ninety percent of patients of systemic sclerosis will have esophageal involvement, but only half of them will be symptomatic. In view of such a high prevalence of esophageal involvement, it may be prudent to start all newly diagnosed cases of systemic sclerosis on proton pump inhibitors to prevent the complications of reflux disease.

In addition, patients who have associated myositis with elevated CPK levels may benefit from steroids to improve the dysphagia.

For more details, please refer to management of gastroesophageal reflux disease.

Gastroesophageal Reflux Disease

The Montreal consensus statement defines gastroesophageal reflux disease (GERD) as a condition which develops when the reflux of gastric content causes troublesome symptoms or complications. GERD prevalence is showing increasing trends throughout the world and especially in Asia.

Symptom complex of GERD has been divided into esophageal and extraesophageal syndromes. Esophageal syndromes include the typical reflux syndrome (heartburn) and reflux chest pain syndromes. Extraesophageal syndromes are classified as those with established associations and those with proposed associations. Established associations include reflux cough, reflux laryngitis, reflux asthma, and reflux dental erosions. Other symptoms with proposed associations are sinusitis, pulmonary fibrosis, recurrent otitis media, and pharyngitis.

Pathophysiology

Transient lower esophageal sphincter relaxation is one of the most important causes for GERD along with hypotensive lower esophageal sphincter. This leads to the disruption of normal anti-reflux barrier at the gastroesophageal junction.

Investigations

Role of endoscopy: The diagnosis of GERD is made on the basis of clinical history alone. Response to antisecretory medication helps in confirming diagnosis;

however, it is not the diagnostic criteria. In subgroup of patients where diagnosis of GERD is unclear; not responding to trial of 4–8 weeks of medication and those with alarm symptoms such as gastrointestinal blood loss, involuntary weight loss, dysphagia, anemia, and age more than 55 years, endoscopy is warranted. The findings on endoscopy are variable ranging from normal to varying degree of esophagitis. GERD is classified as erosive esophagitis (EE) and nonerosive reflux esophagitis [NERD] depending on visible mucosal injury on endosopy (Figs. 5.9 and 5.10). The Los Angeles classification of esophagitis is a widely used grading for severity of esophagitis:

Fig. 5.9 Reflux esophagitis ulcer

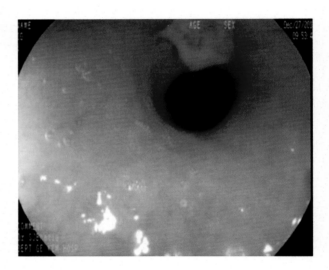

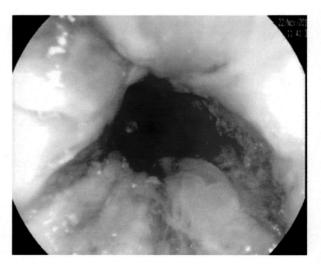

Fig. 5.10 Reflux esophagitis

- Grade A – one or more mucosal breaks each $\leq$5 mm in length
- Grade B – at least one mucosal break >5 mm long, but not continuous between the tops of adjacent mucosal folds
- Grade C – at least one mucosal break that is continuous between the tops of adjacent mucosal folds, but which is not circumferential
- Grade D – mucosal break that involves at least three-fourths of the luminal circumference

However absence of endoscopic features of GERD does not exclude the diagnosis.

Other Investigations

Double contrast barium swallow is not recommended for diagnosis of GERD, but is useful in detection of peptic stricture.

Ambulatory pH monitoring (catheter-based or wireless capsule pHmetry) is useful in confirming diagnosis in persistent symptoms despite trial of PPI in patients with nonerosive reflux esophagitis. It is also used to monitor adequacy of treatment in those with continued symptoms. Transnasally placed catheter and wireless capsule is placed at 5 and 6 cm respectively in distal esophagus above the lower esophageal sphincter. The percentage time the intraesophageal pH remains below 4 is the most useful outcome measured over 24 h pH recording.

Multichannel intraluminal impedance detects intraluminal bolus movement and is usually combined with pHmetry. The basic principle involves measurement of changes in resistance to electric current by pair of metallic rings on the catheter when a bolus passes across. Liquid bolus due to good conductivity lowers the impedance, whereas gas passing across increases impedance. Impedance pHmetry is used for detection of gastroesophageal reflux independent of pH (i.e., both acid and nonacid reflux).It is especially useful in patients with persistent symptoms on acid-suppressive therapy who have normal endoscopic findings.

Esophageal manometry is useful in detecting severe peristaltic dysfunction which may require alteration in the type of wrap to be done during anti-reflux surgery.

Treatment

1. Lifestyle
2. Medical
3. Surgical

Lifestyle modifications include adopting behavior that reduces esophageal acid exposure. Weight loss is recommended for GERD patients who are overweight or have had recent weight gain. Raising the head of the bed by 6–8 in. and avoiding recumbency for 2–3 h after meals have been shown to be of some benefit in nocturnal GERD. Elimination of food items that trigger reflux (fatty or fried food, caffeinated drinks, chocolate, alcohol, acidic or spicy food) is useful in subset of patient. There is lack of evidence on carbonated beverages Small frequent meals are advised in patients with postprandial symptoms.

Medical Treatment

Acid Suppressing Medications

Proton Pump Inhibitor (PPI): Empiric medical therapy with a proton pump inhibitor (PPI) is recommended in patients with typical symptoms of heartburn and regurgitation. PPI therapy for 8 weeks has been associated with superior healing rates and decreased relapse rates as compared with H_2 receptor antagonists (H2RAs) for patients with erosive esophagitis. There are no major differences in efficacy between the different PPIs (omeprazole, lansoprazole, pantoprazole, rabeprazole, and esomeprazole). PPIs should be administered 30–60 min before meal for maximal pH control. PPI therapy is initiated by single-day dosing, before the first meal of the day. In patients with partial response to PPI therapy, increasing the dose to twice daily therapy or switching to a different PPI may provide additional symptom relief. In patients with nighttime symptoms, variable schedules, and/or sleep disturbance, twice daily dosing is found to be effective. Patients whose heartburn has not responded to twice daily PPIs for at least 12 weeks are considered treatment failures and require further evaluation. Maintenance PPI therapy should be administered for GERD patients who continue to have symptoms after PPI is discontinued and in patients with complications including erosive esophagitis and Barrett's esophagus. Long-term PPI therapy is potentially safe though there is a theoretical risk of hypergastrinemia, vitamin B12 and iron deficiency, pneumonia, *Clostridium difficile* colitis, and hip fractures. Short-term PPI usage may increase the risk of community-acquired pneumonia.

H2 Receptor Antagonist (H2RA): H2RA therapy can be used as a maintenance option in patients without erosive disease if patients experience heartburn relief. Bedtime H2RA therapy can be added to daytime PPI therapy in selected patients with objective evidence of nighttime reflux if needed but may be associated with the development of tachyphylaxis after several weeks of use.

Newer drugs that decrease transient lower esophageal sphincter relaxation [tLESR] have been studied with mixed responses. Baclofen GABA[B] agonist decreases tLESR and has been used in refractory GERD; however, neurological side effects of dizziness, drowsiness, and nausea limit its use in clinical practice. Lesogaberan (GABA[B] agonist) does not have CNS side effects but has limited efficacy.

Surgical Treatment

Surgical therapy is a treatment option for long-term therapy in GERD patients. The surgery recommended is laparoscopic fundoplication. Surgical therapy is generally not recommended in patients who do not respond to PPI therapy. Preoperative ambulatory pH monitoring is mandatory in patients without evidence of erosive esophagitis. All patients should undergo preoperative manometry to rule out motility disorder of the esophagus. Surgical therapy is as effective as medical therapy for carefully selected patients with chronic GERD when performed by an experienced surgeon. Obese patients contemplating surgical therapy for GERD should be considered for bariatric surgery. Gastric bypass would be the preferred operation in these patients. The potential side effects of anti-reflux surgery include excessive flatulence, inability to belch, dysphagia, and recurrence of symptoms post surgery (30 % over 5 years).

Endoscopic Treatment: Endoscopic therapy using Stretta or transoral incisionless fundoplication requires further research and presently cannot be recommended as an alternative to medical or traditional surgical therapy.

Benign Esophageal Strictures

The most common form of an esophageal stricture is the peptic stricture, which is sequelae of reflux esophagitis (Fig. 5.11). Other causes include caustic ingestion, Schatzki ring, radiation therapy, anastomotic stricture, post sclerotherapy, pill-induced esophagitis, and eosinophilic esophagitis (Fig. 5.12).

Esophageal strictures are classified as simple and complex stricture.

Simple strictures mainly related to reflux are smooth, straight, and short and can be transversed with the endoscope (<10 mm).

Complex strictures associated with caustic ingestion or radiation induced are long (>2 cm), tortuous, or narrow which precludes passage of normal endoscope. Complex strictures require the use of a guidewire-based system or a balloon dilator. Barium swallow can be performed to define the location and extent of the stricture.

Esophageal dilators used are of three different types. These include bougies filled with mercury or tungsten (e.g., Maloney dilators), wire-guided polyvinyl dilators

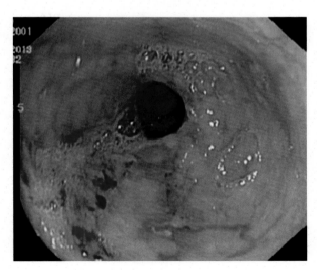

Fig. 5.11 Peptic stricture

Fig. 5.12 Schatzki's ring

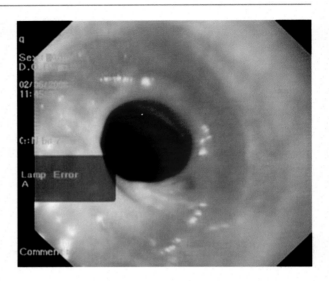

(e.g., Savary-Gilliard [SG] dilators), and through-the-scope (TTS) balloon dilators (controlled radial expansion [CRE™] dilation balloon, with or without guidewire). The latter two dilators are frequently used in practice. The main difference between the dilators is that Savary-Gilliard dilator exerts additional longitudinal force along with radial force which is seen with balloon dilators. Esophageal dilatation is performed under conscious sedation in left lateral decubitus position. The choice of the initial dilator size is based upon the stricture diameter, which can be estimated during radiography or by comparing the stricture to the outer diameter of the endoscope. Usually a guidewire is passed across the stricture through the accessory channel of the endoscope. Endoscope is removed and SG dilators are then passed over the guidewire and dilatation performed under fluoroscopic or endoscopic guidance. In through-the-scope dilators, CRE balloon dilator is passed over the guidewire through the accessory channel. The main complications associated with esophageal dilation include perforation, hemorrhage, and bacteremia. The risk of perforation is minimal if the "rule of three" is applied, meaning that dilation diameters should not increase by more than 3 mm per session. The maximum diameter of 13–14 mm has to be achieved to produce symptomatic relief. Repeated sessions of dilatation may be required which can be done at 5–7 days interval. Treatment with a proton pump inhibitor following dilation may decrease the risk of stricture recurrence. In refractory stricture not amenable to dilatation intralesional steroid has been tried with reasonable success. Recently removable covered metallic and plastic stents are also used.

Esophageal Rings

Esophageal rings are mucosal or muscular structures in distal esophagus that partially or completely compromise the esophageal lumen.

Type A is a muscular ring seen just proximal to the esophagogastric junction. The A (muscular) ring is a symmetrical band of hypertrophied muscle that constricts the tubular esophageal lumen at its junction with the vestibule. It is rare and generally asymptomatic.

Type B (Schatzki ring) is a mucosal ring seen at the squamocolumnar junction. The ring is composed of only mucosa and submucosa; there is no muscularis propria. It is very common and seen in 6–14 % of subjects having a routine upper gastrointestinal series. On barium study, it is seen as a thin membrane constricting the esophageal lumen at the junction of vestibule and gastric cardia. It is seen associated with hiatus hernia hence has been related to gastroesophageal reflux. Most B rings are asymptomatic; however, if the esophageal lumen is <13 mm, it usually leads to intermittent dysphagia.

Endoscopically, an esophageal ring appears as a thin membrane with a concentric smooth contour that projects into the lumen. In symptomatic patients, treatment is aimed at breaking the ring by using the largest diameter of dilator (18–20 mm) and a short course of postdilation anti-reflux therapy to reduce the need of repeat dilation. Endoscopic electrosurgical incision with needle knife can be used in refractory cases.

Esophageal Webs

Esophageal webs are developmental anomalies commonly seen in cervical esophagus and midesophagus. Esophageal webs protrude from the anterior wall, extending laterally but not to the posterior wall and unlike rings rarely encircle the lumen. Webs are thin mucosal layer covered with squamous epithelium. Most common presentation is dysphagia mainly to solids. Esophageal webs are diagnosed by videofluoroscopy and are best demonstrated on an esophagogram with the lateral view. Endoscopically, it appears as a thin membrane protruding in the esophageal lumen. Webs respond well to esophageal bougienage.

Esophageal web associated with iron-deficiency anemia and dysphagia forms the triad seen in Plummer-Vinson syndrome or Paterson-Kelly syndrome mainly seen in adult females. These patients are at increased risk of esophageal cancer. Treatment of iron deficiency itself may lead to resolution of dysphagia as well as disappearance of webs.

Eosinophilic Esophagitis (EoE)

EoE is a chronic inflammatory condition defined by symptoms of esophageal dysfunction, an eosinophilic infiltrate in the esophageal epithelium, and the absence of other potential causes of eosinophilia. The diagnostic criteria for EoE include (1) symptoms related to esophageal dysfunction, (2) peak value of >15 eosinophil/hpf, (3) eosinophilia limited to the esophagus, (4) and other causes of esophageal eosinophilia excluded, particularly PPI-responsive esophageal eosinophilia.

EoE is thought to be an immune-mediated disorder in which food or environmental antigens stimulate an inflammatory response which leads to production of cytokines (IL-4, 5, and 13, eotaxin 3) leading to recruitment of eosinophils in esophagus.

EoE is seen most commonly before the age of 40 years. It is the cause of heartburn in 1–8 % of patients with PPI-refractory symptoms of GERD. In adolescent and adults, the common presentation is dysphagia and food impaction. Nonspecific symptoms of feeding intolerance, failure to thrive, nausea, vomiting, and regurgitation may be seen in younger children.

Endoscopic appearance is variable and includes fixed or transient esophageal rings (feline esophagus), narrow-caliber esophagus, strictures, linear furrows, mucosal pallor, congestion, or decreased vascularityand white plaques or exudates and fragile esophageal mucosa, termed crepe paper mucosa, where a tear occurs with passage of the endoscope (Fig. 5.13). Esophagus may also appear normal in 7–10 % of patients. At least 2–4 biopsy is taken from distal and proximal esophagus to maximize the diagnosis. On biopsy, eosinophilic infiltrate in the esophageal epithelium with >15 eosinophils/hpf suggests the diagnosis of EoE. Associated histopathologic features of EoE include eosinophil degranulation; eosinophil microabscesses, defined by clusters of >4 eosinophils; basal zone hyperplasia or rete peg elongation; spongiosis; and fibrosis of the lamina propria.

Treatment includes three general categories termed as "the three D's": drugs, diet, and dilation. Drugs like topical steroids are the first-line agents as they are well tolerated. Topical steroids used are swallowed fluticasone 440 mcg twice daily for at least 6 weeks or swallowed budesonide 1–2 mg for 3 months. Unfortunately, when topical or systemic corticosteroids are discontinued, the disease generally reappears. Other drugs like leukotriene antagonists (montelukast) and mast cell stabilizers are reserved as a second-line agent in selected cases. Immunomodulators (azathioprine) and recently anti-IL-5 (mepolizumab) are in

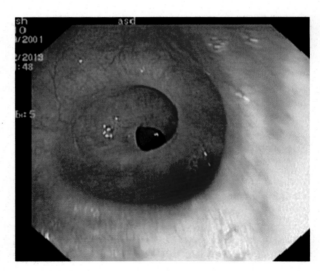

Fig. 5.13 Eosinophilic esophagitis

experimental stages in treatment of EoE. Systemic steroids could be considered if symptoms are severe or need to be treated quickly because of malnutrition.

Dietary elimination of allergenic diet also can be used because food allergens have been suggested to contribute to the pathogenesis of EoE. There are three general strategies for dietary elimination in EoE: elemental diet, six-food elimination diet (SFED), and targeted elimination diet. Elemental diet is composed of amino acids, basic carbohydrates, and medium chain triglycerides. However, elemental formulas are expensive and unpalatable. Six-food elimination diet was developed to increase compliance and acceptability. SFED eliminates six of the most common food allergens: milk, eggs, wheat, soy, seafood, and nuts. Dilatation is used when medical treatment fails for esophageal stricture, esophageal narrowing, or persistent fixed rings causing dysphagia. However, risk of perforation is high.

Lymphocytic Esophagitis

Lymphocytic esophagitis is described as increase numbers of infiltrating intraepithelial lymphocytes, which expressed CD3, CD4, and CD8 markers. It is characterized by dense lymphocytic infiltrates (at least >20/hpf) in the peripapillary esophageal squamous mucosa and marked spongiosis (edema of the intercellular spaces) in the absence of significant numbers of neutrophils or eosinophils. Lymphocytic esophagitis affects predominantly older women and presents with dysphagia, odynophagia, and motility disorders. Endoscopic features seen were similar to EoE in two-thirds of the patients which included felinization with furrows, whitish plaques, and strictures.

Recently narrow band imaging with magnifying endoscopy (NBI-ME) has shown the presence of the following three features: 1) beige discoloration of mucosa, 2)increased and congested intrapapillary capillary loop and 3)invisibility of submucosal vascularity which aid in the diagnosis of Lymphocytic and Eosinophilic esophagitis and differentiates from GERD.

Infectious Esophagitis

Infections of the esophagus present with acute dysphagia, odynophagia, and chest pain.

Esophageal Candidiasis

Esophageal candidiasis is more commonly seen in immunodeficiency disorders like diabetes mellitus, chronic renal failure, alcoholism and AIDS, and individuals on steroids and chemotherapeutic agents. In achalasia and scleroderma due to stasis of food, esophageal candidiasis can occur. Endoscopy reveals raised white pseudomembranous plaques with mucosal erythema (Fig. 5.14). In severe cases, confluent linear and nodular plaques with underlying ulcerations may be present. Esophageal candidiasis can be confirmed by brush cytology smear showing

Fig. 5.14 Esophageal
candidiasis

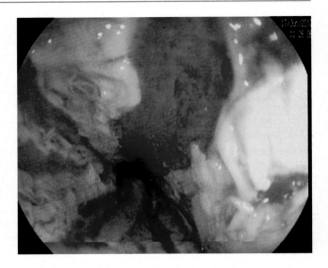

Fig. 5.15 CMV ulcer

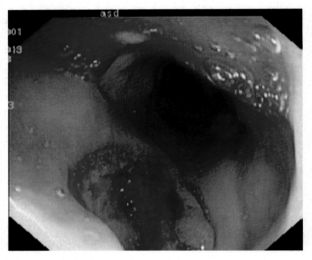

hyphae. Treatment consists of 10–20 mL of oral nystatin (100,000 units/mL) 6 hourly, oral clotrimazole (10 mg 6 hourly), or fluconazole 100 mg per day for 7 days. Caspofungin can be used for treatment if resistance to antifungal medication is demonstrated.

Viral Esophagitis

Cytomegalovirus esophagitis occurs only in the immunocompromised host. Endoscopy shows serpiginous ulcers which are large and deep with surrounding normal mucosa (Fig. 5.15). Biopsy should be taken from the center of the ulcer and reveals intranuclear and small cytoplasmic inclusion bodies. Treatment consists of ganciclovir (5 mg/kg 12 hourly) for few weeks. Valganciclovir or foscarnet can also be used till healing of ulcer as alternative treatment.

Herpes simplex virus (HSV) esophagitis is caused by HSV 1 and 2. On endoscopy, small vesicles and discrete punched-out lesions are seen and it may proceed to confluent ulcers. Biopsy from edge of the ulcer may show ballooning degeneration, ground-glass change in nuclei with eosinophilic inclusions (Cowdry type A), and giant cell formation. Treatment consists of acyclovir (400 mg orally five times a day for 14–21 days) or valacyclovir (1 g three times a day for 7 days). Varicella-zoster virus occasionally produces esophagitis in children with chicken pox and adults with herpes zoster with lesion similar to HSV. Higher dose of acyclovir is used in varicella infection.

Esophageal Tuberculosis

Esophageal tuberculosis is rare but appears to be increasing specially in immuno-compromised patients. It is almost always due to contiguous spread from the lung or mediastinal lymph nodes, and very few isolated primary esophageal tuberculosis has been reported. Endoscopy shows deep, large, or irregular ulcers or tracheo-esophageal fistulous opening. Biopsy from the ulcer or the underlying lymph node might help in confirming the diagnosis. Antituberculosis drugs are used for treatment. Tracheoesophageal fistula may require surgical treatment if not healing with antituberculosis treatment.

Pill Esophagitis

Pill-induced esophageal injury results from damage due to ingestion of certain medications which cause injury by either production of caustic solution, hyperosmolar solution, or direct drug damage. The common drugs implicated are tetracycline, doxycycline, potassium chloride, nonsteroidal anti-inflammatory drugs, alendronate, and ferrous sulfate. The most common location of pill-induced esophagitis is in the midesophagus at the crossing of aorta or carina. Endoscopy may reveal an ulcer or diffuse esophagitis. Treatment consists of withdrawal of the offending drug and use of proton pump inhibitors along with viscous lignocaine.

Corrosive Injury to Esophagus

Corrosive damage to esophagus occurs following ingestion of strong alkali or acid. Severity of injury depends on several factors like quantity, substance pH, physical state, tissue contact time, and concentration. Lesser damage occurs with acids than alkali. Acids causes coagulative necrosis which limits its penetration, and also due to its offensive smells, lesser amount is ingested, whereas alkali causes liquefactive necrosis and thrombosis of the vessel wall leading to deeper penetration and damage. In the esophagus, corrosives pool at the post-cricoid area, level of aortic arch, tracheal bifurcation, and lower esophageal sphincter. These are common locations for strictures. Assessment of the severity of damage is most important after resuscitation of the patient. Endoscopy can be performed at the earliest within 72 h after ruling out perforation by imaging. Endoscopic grading is helpful in management and prognostication. Endoscopic grading of caustic injury is as follows:

Grade	Endoscopic findings
I	Edema and erythema
IIA	Hemorrhage, erosions, blisters, ulcers with exudate
IIB	Circumferential ulceration
III	Multiple deep ulcers with brown, black, or gray discoloration
IV	Perforation

Patients of Grade I or IIA injury can be started on oral liquids by 48 h and can be discharged early. Patients with Grade IIB injury and III injury should be admitted to an intensive care unit and managed with intravenous fluid resuscitation and close monitoring for evidence of perforation. A nasojejunal tube can be placed over a guidewire during endoscopy; this serves as a route for maintaining nutrition and also provides a lumen for dilatation in future as these patients are prone to develop strictures (Fig. 5.16). Strictures most commonly develop after 6–8 weeks of caustic ingestion. Corrosive stricture requires more sessions of dilatation as compared to noncorrosive strictures (Fig. 5.17). Intralesional steroid and self-expanding removable stents can be used in refractory strictures. Esophageal squamous cell carcinoma is a potential long-term complication of corrosive injury.

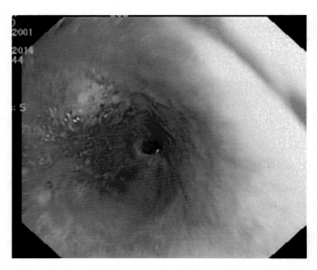

Fig. 5.16 Corrosive stricture

Fig. 5.17 Post-dilatation corrosive stricture

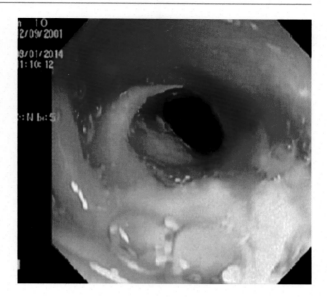

Radiation Injury to Esophagus

Early injury is seen within 2–3 week of radiation therapy of thoracic and upper abdominal malignancies. Endoscopically, mucositis and ulceration may be observed. It usually is managed by mediations like topical anesthetics, oral analgesics, and gastric antisecretory drugs. Late complications such as benign stricture and persistent ulceration may occur months to years following treatment and are dose related. The management of late esophageal radiation stricture consists of endoscopic dilatation.

Foreign Bodies and Food Impaction

Foreign body ingestion is mainly seen in children particularly in age group of 6 months to 3 years and psychiatric patients. Coins, marbles, small toys, crayons, nails, and pins are the most common foreign bodies that are ingested.

The posterior pharynx is the first area in which foreign bodies may become entrapped. In esophagus food boluses and foreign bodies become lodged in areas of normal anatomical narrowing part of the esophagus.

Radiological imaging like plain film of X-ray (anteroposterior and lateral) can be done to determine the presence, type, number, and location of foreign objects present. Endoscopy confirms foreign boy ingestion and also used for retrieval of foreign bodies with accessories like grasping forceps, retrieval nets, and dormia basket (Fig. 5.18). Sharp objects may require transparent hood or caps to withdraw the object into it before removal to prevent mucosal damage.

Fig. 5.18 Foreign body
esophagus

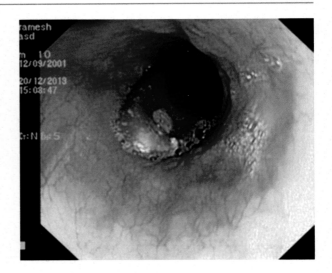

Food impactions most commonly occur in adults in their fourth or fifth decade of life. It occurs mainly with an underlying esophageal pathology like peptic stricture, Schatzki ring, eosinophilic esophagitis, postsurgical altered anatomy, or motility disorders. Fish bone, meat, and chicken are the common food which gets impacted.

The primary method to treat food impaction is the push method in which the impacted food is pushed into the stomach with the endoscope. If a large food bolus is impacted, it can be broken with endoscopic accessories before being pushed into the stomach.

Esophageal Cancer

Esophageal carcinoma is the seventh most common cause of cancer mortality worldwide. Overall esophageal carcinoma carries a poor prognosis with 5-year survival of 19 %. The most common esophageal cancers are squamous cell cancer (SCC) and adenocarcinoma. Squamous cell cancer is the commonest type of esophageal carcinoma worldwide. Esophageal cancers occur most commonly in the sixth and seventh decade. Esophageal cancers are more commonly seen in males than females having male to female ratio of 3–4:1. Smoking and alcohol are major risk factors for SCC, while Barrett's esophagus, obesity, and smoking are the risk factors for adenocarcinoma. Preexisting esophageal disease like achalasia, Plummer-Vinson syndrome, tylosis, caustic and radiation strictures, and history of aerodigestive cancers increases risk of squamous cell cancer. Dysphagia initially to solids eventually progressing to include liquids and weight loss of short duration are the most common symptoms. Other symptoms are odynophagia, hematemesis retrosternal pain, hoarseness of voice, and bone pain due to metastasis. Esophagorespiratory fistula develops in approximately 5–15 % of all patients with advanced esophageal cancer.

Fig. 5.19 Esophageal
cancer

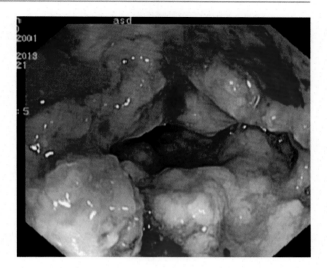

Diagnosis can be done by endoscopy and biopsy. Barium swallow shows rat tail-like narrowing or filling defect with irregular mucosa.

On endoscopy, superficial plaques, nodules, or ulcerations are seen in early stages, and proliferative, ulcerated, or ulceroproliferative masses or strictures are seen in advanced lesions (Fig. 5.19). Biopsy is performed for confirming the malignancy, and at least 6–8 biopsy specimens are usually taken which increases the diagnostic yield to 98 %. In strictures, complete visualization and sampling of the obstructing malignancy is difficult; brush cytology can improve the diagnostic accuracy by 20 % in such cases. Transoral or transnasal ultrathin endoscopes also may be used for obstructing malignancies to visualize the extent and length of the tumor. The sensitivity of detecting early stage carcinoma may be improved by targeted biopsies using enhanced mucosal imaging like chromoendoscopy (dye-based staining) and narrow band imaging (using blue and green light). However, further studies are required for enhanced mucosal imaging technique.

Staging of Esophageal Malignancies

CT scan and endosonography (EUS) are used in staging of tumor. CT scan is typically the initial staging modality, once a diagnosis has been established by endoscopy. CT is valuable in detecting metastatic disease in the liver, lungs, and periaortic lymph nodes. CT has a reasonable accuracy in detecting invasion of mediastinal structures in locally advanced tumors and has accuracy rates of up to 90 % in detecting aortic, tracheobronchial, and pericardial invasion. However, the constituent layers of the esophageal wall cannot be easily differentiated from each other; hence, CT has poor accuracy (50–60 %) in assessing local tumor stage.

PET is more sensitive and specific than CT for detecting distant metastases in patients with esophageal carcinoma. However, the sensitivity of FDG PET for detecting locoregional disease is low and inferior to EUS.

Role of Endoscopic Ultrasound (EUS) in Esophageal Malignancies

Endoscopic ultrasound is the modality of choice for locoregional tumor staging with accuracy of up to 90 %. EUS provides an assessment of the tumor stage. EUS accurately detects the T staging as it delineates all the five layers of the esophagus and hence correctly detects the depth of invasion of the tumor. EUS also helps in preoperative staging of lymph nodes. Endosonographic criteria that are suggestive of malignant involvement of visible lymph nodes include a width greater than 10 mm, round shape, smooth border, and echo-poor pattern. EUS-guided fine needle aspiration of lymph node can improve the accuracy of N staging by providing cytology for confirmation of meta-static lesion with sensitivity of 90 %. In stenotic tumor, EUS has its limitation due to the size of the echoendoscope; however, miniprobes can be used in such circumstances.

AmericanJoint Committee on Cancer Staging System for cancers of the esophagus

Tumor node metastasis definitions
Primary tumor (T)
TX: primary tumor cannot be assessed
T0: no evidence of primary tumor
Tis: carcinoma in situ (T1a or T1m)
T1: tumor invades lamina propria or submucosa (T1b, or T1sm)
T2: tumor invades muscularis propria
T3: tumor invades adventitia
T4: tumor invades adjacent structures
Regional lymph nodes (N)
NX: regional lymph nodes cannot be assessed
N0: no regional lymph node metastasis
N1: regional lymph node metastasis
Distant metastasis (M)
MX: distant metastasis cannot be assessed
M0: no distant metastasis
M1: distant metastasis
Tumors of the lower thoracic esophagus:
M1a: metastasis in celiac lymph nodes
M1b: other distant metastasis
Tumors of the midthoracic esophagus:
M1a: not applicable
M1b: nonregional lymph nodes and/or other distant metastasis

Tumor node metastasis definitions
Tumors of the upper thoracic esophagus:
M1a: metastasis in cervical nodes
M1b: other distant metastasis

AJCC stage groupings
Stage 0
Tis, N0, M0
Stage I
T1, N0, M0
Stage IIA
T2, N0, M0
T3, N0, M0
Stage IIB
T1, N1, M0
T2, N1, M0
Stage III
T3, N1, M0
T4, any N, M0
Stage IV
Any T, any N, M1
Stage IVA
Any T, any N, M1a
Stage IVB
Any T, any N, M1b

The prognosis for patients with esophageal carcinoma is poor. Primary treatment modalities comprise resection of the primary tumor, chemotherapy, and radiotherapy. The treatment of esophageal cancer varies according to the stage of cancer.

Endoscopic therapy (e.g., mucosal resection or submucosal dissection) can be considered for Tis and Stage I: T1a N0 (on EUS). Initial surgery can be considered for T1b and any N. In stage II–III neoadjuvant chemoradiation is followed by surgery (trimodality therapy). In stage IV chemotherapy or symptomatic and supportive care is given.

Role of Endoscopy in Treatment of Esophageal Malignancy

Endoscopic therapy for esophageal cancer can be categorized broadly as therapy with curative intent or therapy to palliate symptoms. Accurate staging of early cancers is required if curative treatment is planned. Stage T1a malignancies include lesions confined to the mucosa: M1 (intraepithelial), M2 (lamina propria invasion), or M3 (muscularis mucosa invasion). Submucosal or T1b malignancies are classified into Sm1 (superficial submucosa invasion), Sm2 (invasion to center of submucosa), or Sm3 (invasion to deep submucosa).

Endoscopic therapy of early stage esophageal cancer can be divided broadly into resection and ablation techniques. The advantage of resection over ablation therapy is the availability of large tissue specimens for pathologic diagnosis and accurate cancer staging.

Endoscopic mucosal resection (EMR) and endoscopic submucosal dissection (ESD) can be performed in esophageal cancer limited to mucosa. EMR is indicated for T1a lesions and may be used for flat Barrett's esophagus with high-grade dysplasia. EMR commonly is performed using a "suck and cut" method in which the endoscopist elevates the dysplastic area by injecting fluid into the submucosa, after which the elevated mucosa is suctioned into a cap that fits over the tip of the endoscope, and polypectomy snare is then deployed around the suctioned area to remove it. Another variation of the "band and snare" method uses an endoscopic variceal ligating device to deploy elastic bands around the suctioned mucosal segment. It does not require prior submucosal fluid injection and the banded segment is removed using a polypectomy snare. ESD can be used in similar situations but is preferred to EMR for large areas of dysplasia (>2 cm) or T1b malignancies (i.e., confined to the submucosa). ESD involves a deeper and larger resection of the esophageal wall by dissecting the submucosal connective tissue just beneath the target lesion from the underlying muscle layer using the hook knife or other electrocautery devices. However, ESD requires high level of expertise on the part of the endoscopist. EMR successfully eradicates 91–98 % of T1a cancers. Potential complications of EMR are bleeding, perforation, and stricture formation.

Ablation techniques for intramucosal carcinoma include photodynamic therapy (PDT), cryotherapy, argon plasma coagulation (APC), heater probe treatment, and radiofrequency ablation (RFA). However, expertise is required to perform these techniques and currently this is limited to a few clinicians. Also the long-term outcome and recurrence after these techniques is under evaluation and hence these techniques are not recommended at present for treatment of esophageal cancer.

In operable cases, different surgical techniques have been used for primary management of esophageal cancer. Transhiatal esophagectomy and Ivor-Lewis transthoracic esophagectomy are the most common surgeries performed. Esophageal cancers are inoperable if metastasis to N_2 (celiac, cervical, supraclavicular) nodes or solid organs (e.g., liver, lung) or invasion of adjacent structures (e.g., recurrent laryngeal nerve, tracheobronchial tree, aorta, pericardium) is present.

There are several endoscopic palliative measures for dysphagia in inoperable cases. Endoscopic options for palliation include dilation, stenting, chemical or ablative debulking, and enteral feeding. Esophageal stenting with self-expandable metal stent (partially and fully covered SEMS) are preferred for palliation of dysphagia and in tracheoesophageal fistula. A variety of esophageal SEMSs are commercially available (Wallstent, Ultraflex, Z stent, Niti S stent, Anti-reflux Dua stent); however, there are no differences among the various stents in palliating malignant dysphagia. Stent complications include intolerable chest pain, perforation, migration, tumor, ingrowth, bleeding, and fistula formation. Esophageal dilatation can be performed using polyvinyl dilator or through-the-scope balloon dilator. Malignant strictures can be dilated up to 14–16 mm in repeated sessions but with increased risk of perforation and is usually not done. Endoscopic techniques also may be used to debulk an inoperable, obstructing tumor using chemical debulking, laser ablation, and PDT.

Extrinsic Compression of Esophagus

Mediastinal tumor, aberrant subclavian artery, and lymph nodes cause extrinsic compression of the esophagus. On endoscopy luminal narrowing is noted with overlying mucosa being normal.

Submucosal tumor of the esophagus like gastrointestinal tumor, lipoma, and granulosa cell tumor also appears as elevated lesions in the esophagus. EUS is useful for evaluation and biopsy of mediastinal lymph nodes.

Radiological Diagnosis in Swallowing Disorders

Devaki V. Dewan

Definition

Dysphagia or difficulty swallowing is a comprehensive term used to describe the inability to propel the food bolus from the mouth to the stomach.

Peristalsis

Peristalsis refers to the coordinated wave of contractions that occurs from the proximal to distal extent of the esophagus resulting in propulsion of a food bolus from the proximal esophagus to the stomach. This results from progressive and coordinated contraction of the longitudinal and circular esophageal musculature sequentially from the proximal to the distal esophagus.

Primary peristalsis is a wave of contractions which occur at a set speed and is triggered by the swallowing center located in the medulla. Secondary peristalsis results from esophageal distension caused by a bolus of food, causing contraction above and relaxation below the bolus, allowing for the distal transfer of the food bolus along the esophagus. Appropriately functioning primary and secondary peristalses result in smooth transit of a food bolus from the oropharynx to the stomach. Tertiary contractions on the other hand are non-physiologic uncoordinated contractions that may occur simultaneously in different parts of the esophagus and in no particular time sequence, impeding progression of the food bolus and resulting in dysphagia (Fig. 6.1).

D.V. Dewan, MD
Radiology and Imaging, Radiology Associates of Clearwater,
1106 Druid Rd. S., Suite 302, Clearwater, FL 33756, USA
e-mail: devaki@dewan.pro

© Springer India 2015
G. Mankekar (ed.), *Swallowing – Physiology, Disorders, Diagnosis and Therapy*,
DOI 10.1007/978-81-322-2419-8_6

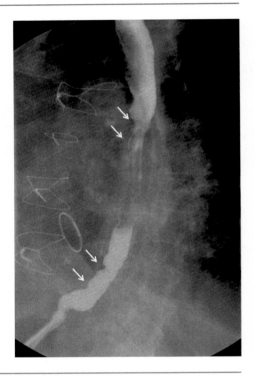

Fig. 6.1 Tertiary contraction of the esophagus. Uncoordinated contractions are seen in the mid to distal esophagus (*arrows*)

Etiology

Dysphagia may be caused (Table 6.1) by a neurological deficit, which is temporary with expected recovery, such as seen with a transient ischemic attack (TIA) or a cerebrovascular accident (CVA) [1], progressive as in neuromuscular conditions such as scleroderma or multiple sclerosis, or more static conditions which include the post polio syndrome. In scleroderma, the esophageal smooth muscle is replaced by fibrous tissue resulting in diminished peristaltic activity and resultant dysphagia (Fig. 6.2). Esophageal dysmotility may be seen in the elderly where it is known as presbyesophagus. In this condition, there is inefficient propulsion of the food bolus due to tertiary contractions in the esophagus. These result in uncoordinated contractions of the esophagus with resultant dysphagia and at times heartburn. Cognitive disability or psychosis may also result in dysphagia. Certain radiological tests are useful in distinguishing between the various abnormalities.

Structural or obstructive causes of dysphagia can be accurately diagnosed with radiological tests. These include esophageal webs, diverticula, Schatzki rings, strictures, neoplasms, or an obstructed foreign body. Esophageal diverticula are outpouchings of the esophageal wall that occur at sites of anatomic weakness in the hypopharynx or the cervical esophagus adjacent to the cricopharyngeus muscle [2]. Achalasia is a condition wherein both neurological and obstructive etiologies come into play [3] (Fig. 6.3a, b). A Schatzki ring is a mucosal ring in the distal esophagus at the squamo-columnar junction. This may or may not be symptomatic based on its luminal diameter. Schatzki rings are most often responsible for episodic dysphagia to solid foods. The

Table 6.1 Causes of
dysphagia

Neurological	TIA/CVA
	Scleroderma
	Multiple sclerosis
	Post polio syndrome
	Muscular dystrophy
	Presbyesophagus
	Achalasia
Obstructive	Parapharyngeal/peritonsillar abscess
	Esophagitis
	Esophageal diverticula
	Esophageal web and Schatzki ring
	Benign or malignant esophageal stricture
	Primary or secondary achalasia
	Hiatal hernia

Fig. 6.2 Scleroderma.
Featureless esophagus due to
markedly diminished
peristaltic activity

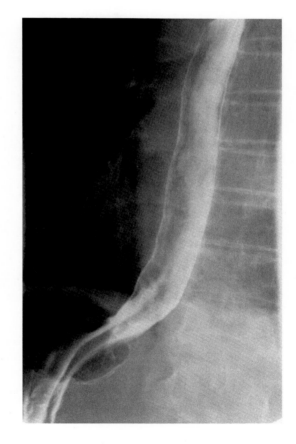

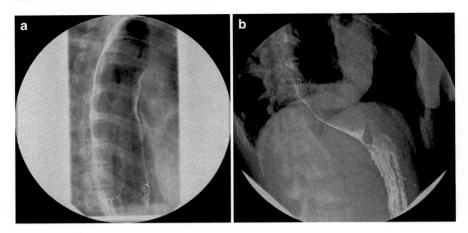

Fig. 6.3 Achalasia (**a**, **b**). The proximal and mid esophagus during a double-contrast esophagram (**a**) shows an overly distended esophagus. A bird beak appearance of the distal esophagus (**b**) due to non-relaxation of the distal esophageal sphincter

Fig. 6.4 Schatzki ring.
A shelf-like indentation in the
distal esophagus (*curved
arrows*) which was
symptomatic in this patient
due to significant narrowing
of the esophageal lumen

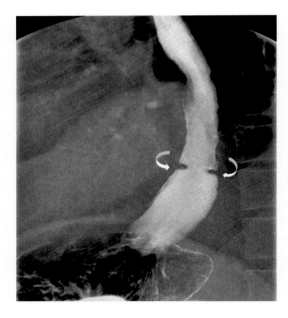

pathogenesis is unknown and proposed theories include congenital, developmental, and post inflammatory etiologies (Fig. 6.4) [4]. An esophageal web occurs in the proximal esophagus and is usually anterior in location and more often eccentric.

The type of examination and frequency or need for a repeat evaluation would depend upon the pathology suspected clinically and subsequently diagnosed radiologically.

Gamut of Imaging Tests Available in the Evaluation of Dysphagia [5]

I. Fluoroscopic tests
   1. Dynamic assessment: videofluoroscopic swallowing study (VSS) also known as the modified barium swallow (MVS)
   2. Barium swallow and esophagogram
II. CT scan of the neck and chest
III. MRI of the neck

Patient Preparation for the Radiological Examination

The patient is advised to stay NPO after midnight prior to a fluoroscopic test. The patient has to be NPO for 4–6 h prior to a CT scan or MRI performed with intravenous contrast. To alleviate anxiety and to improve patient participation and cooperation, it is advisable that the referring clinician inform the patient of the nature and benefit of the examination. Any contraindications or limitations such as radiographic contrast allergy or renal dysfunction are sought out in a screening questionnaire at the time of scheduling the examination. In cases of minor contrast allergy, the patient would be pretreated with oral prednisone and diphenhydramine. At our facilities we use a 16-h pretreatment protocol where the patient receives 50 mg oral prednisone at 8 h intervals with the last dose of prednisone taken along with 50 mg diphenhydramine within 30 min of contrast administration. When the patient arrives in the radiology department, he/she is then informed in detail about the procedure. Patient participation with regard to holding still is communicated to the patient by the radiology technologist just prior to the procedure being performed and again at the precise moment when the patient is needed to comply with this request.

Fluoroscopic Tests

Videofluoroscopic Swallowing Study (VSS)
Procedure: The patient is positioned seated facing laterally facing the speech pathologist (Fig. 6.5). Various consistencies of liquid barium and barium-coated solid foods are used to test the patient's swallowing ability. This test is performed in conjunction with the speech and swallowing therapist, thereby allowing the therapist the opportunity to assess the patient for the potential usefulness of and the type of swallowing therapy to be utilized.

The following conditions may be diagnosed with this test:
Oropharyngeal incoordination.
Laryngeal vestibular penetration or frank aspiration (Fig. 6.6).
If aspiration is detected, if silent or with elicitation of a cough reflex
Objective severity of dysphagia
Lack of elevation of the larynx and closure of the airway, for example, after surgery for head and neck carcinoma

Fig. 6.5 Patient positioned
facing the speech pathologist
with the image intensifier
lateral to the patient so as to
obtain a lateral view of the
oral cavity and pharynx
during VSS

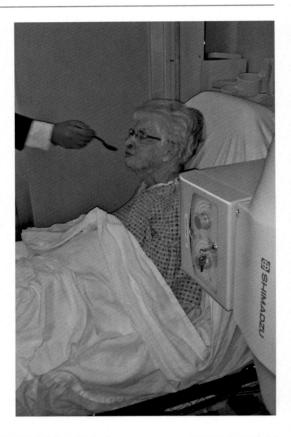

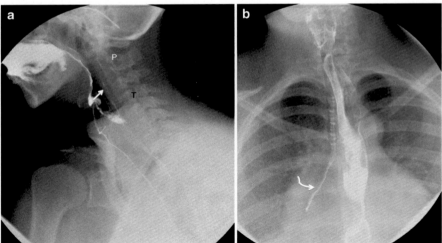

Fig. 6.6 Aspiration. Lateral view (**a**) of the pharynx and larynx with aspiration of barium which
has penetration below the level of the vocal cords (*arrow*). *P* pyriform fossa, *T* subglottic trachea.
AP view of the neck and chest (**b**) shows aspiration of barium into the right main and lower lobe
bronchus (*curved arrow*)

Barium Swallow with Esophagogram

Procedure: Thick barium (barium sulfate suspension 250 w/v) is given orally to the patient with him standing, in order to assess the oropharynx and hypopharynx. This step also allows the evaluation for any aspiration prior to continuing on with the rest of the examination. The patient then swallows effervescent granules chased with small sips of water, following which with thick barium. The air produced by the swallowed granules and the barium create a double contrast within the esophagus with demonstration of excellent mucosal detail of the esophageal lining. This is important in the assessment of mucosal irregularities or ulcerations. Conditions such as reflux esophagitis (Fig. 6.7) or the nature of a stricture, namely, irregular or smoothly contoured, may come to light at this stage of the examination. The patient is now guided into an RAO position on the fluoroscopic table (Fig. 6.8). He drinks thin barium (barium sulfate suspension 70 w/v) in continuous sips with a wide bore straw, so as to maximally distend the esophagus. The position of the patient who is lying on the table in an RAO position allows for the assessment of true peristaltic activity, having eliminated the influence of gravity.

The relevant normal anatomy of the pharynx and esophagus as it appears on the barium swallow and esophagogram is reviewed [6]. The pharynx comprises of the oropharynx and hypopharynx which are separated by the pharyngoepiglottic fold. The cricopharyngeus muscle marks the beginning of the esophagus. In the normal pharynx, one sees symmetric valleculae and pyriform sinuses. The valecullae are

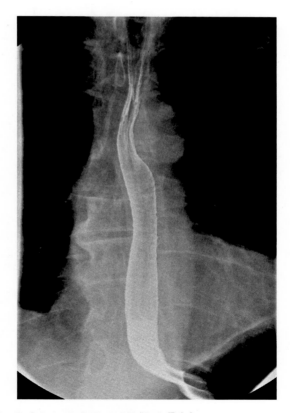

Fig. 6.7 Esophagitis. Punctate foci of barium pooling within the esophageal mucosa in a patient with reflux esophagitis

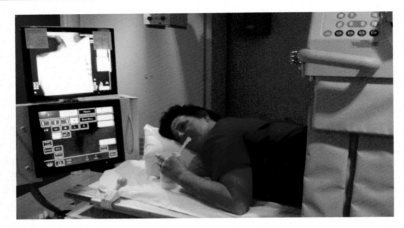

Fig. 6.8 RAO position during a single-contrast esophagram. The patient drinks thin barium from a wide bore straw while lying in this prone oblique position

Fig. 6.9 Normal pharyngeal anatomy. A small amount of barium is seen pooling within the valleculae (*V*) which appear symmetric. The valecullae are separated by the median glossoepiglottic fold (*solid straight arrows*). Barium also outlines the pyriform sinuses (*P*). The tongue base is outlined (*thin white arrows*)

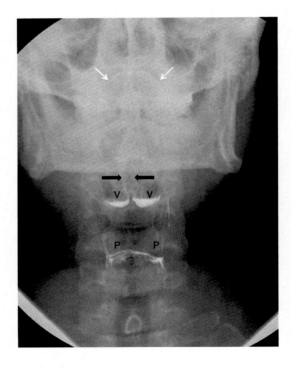

recesses between the tongue base and epiglottis, divided by the median glossoepi-glottic fold (Fig. 6.9). The pyriform sinuses are lateral recesses arising from the lateral laryngeal walls and extending into the hypopharynx bilaterally. The normal esophagus is smoothly contoured, extending from the cricopharyngeus muscle at the C5–C6 levels to the gastroesophageal junction. Smooth linear mucosal folds are observed in a normal esophagus. Saccular termination of the esophagus is physio-logic and is termed the esophageal vestibule (Fig. 6.10a–c).

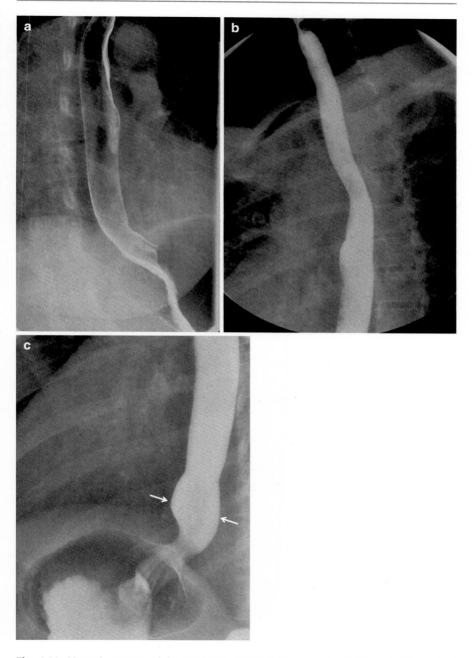

Fig. 6.10 Normal anatomy of the esophagus. (**a**) Normal mucosal relief in a double-contrast esophagram. (**b**) Uniformly distended esophagram during a single-contrast esophagram. (**c**) Appearance of the esophageal ampula which is the normal distended distal portion of the esophagus (*arrows*)

This test pinpoints the location of a lesion, from the tongue base to the gastrointestinal junction. It also assesses the distensibility of the esophagus at the site of a stricture which is useful information to aid in distinguishing benign from malignant strictures. This is a very useful test to evaluate the success of a dilatation procedure for a benign esophageal stricture and should the patient's symptoms recur to evaluate the need for repeat intervention.

Differentiating between a fixed peptic stricture (Fig. 6.11) and lack of relaxation of the distal esophageal sphincter in cases of achalasia (Fig. 6.3b) may be confidently accomplished with the help of the esophagram [7].

We will now discuss some of the conditions that can be identified using barium swallow and esophagram tests. Lesions at the tongue base, valleculae, or pyriform sinuses cause high dysphagia. Tongue base or vallecular lesions may be detected by flexible endoscopy in the otolaryngologist's office. However, lesions of the valleculae or pyriform sinuses may at times be first picked up on a barium swallow, obtained by the primary care physician for a patient presenting with early symptoms of dysphagia.

There are several entities that may cause extrinsic compression on the esophagus and thereby result in symptoms of dysphagia. A hypertrophied cricopharyngeus muscle causes indentation of the posterior esophageal wall and thereby results in difficulty swallowing (Fig. 6.12). Cervical vertebral osteophytes along the

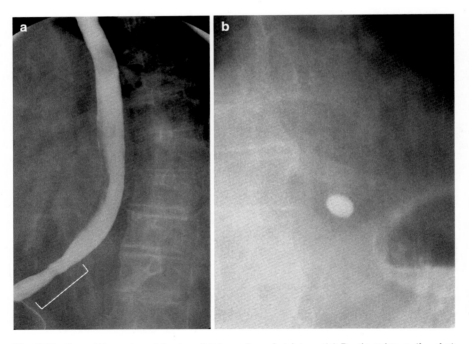

Fig. 6.11 Smoothly contoured benign distal esophageal stricture. (**a**) Peptic stricture (*bracket*) caused as a result of scarring and fibrosis due to long-standing reflux esophagitis. (**b**) Holdup of a barium tablet at the stricture

Fig. 6.12 Indentation of a hypertrophied cricopharyngeus muscle (*solid arrow*) resulting in narrowing of the lumen of the cervical esophagus.

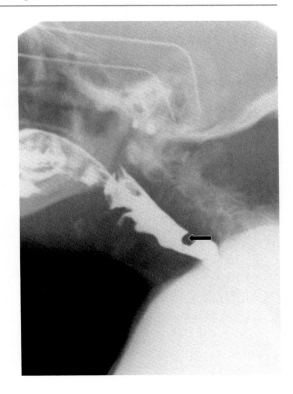

anterior margins of the vertebral bodies most commonly occur at the C5 to C7 levels. The presence of osteophytes allows less room for esophageal distention when the food bolus approaches that segment of the esophagus (Fig. 6.13a, b). In the mediastinum, an ectasia or aneurysm of the aorta may cause extrinsic compression on the thoracic portion of the esophagus (Fig. 6.14). Mediastinal fibrosis due to a variety of causes including post-radiation fibrosis or following chronic inflammatory disease may limit the distensibility of the thoracic esophagus resulting in dysphagia of varying degrees.

Esophageal diverticula are outpouching of the esophageal wall. They occur at sites of anatomic weakness in the hypopharynx or cervical esophagus, adjacent to the cricopharyngeus muscle [2, 6]. A Zenker's diverticulum (Fig. 6.15) is a posterior esophageal diverticulum that occurs along the mid-posterior esophageal wall, just superior to the cricopharyngeus muscle. This is often seen in patients who have a prominent cricopharyngeus muscle. A Killian-Jamieson diverticulum occurs along the anterolateral wall of the cervical esophagus and is inferior to the cricopharyngeus muscle (Fig. 6.16a, b). Radiological findings help distinguish between these diverticula based not only on the posterior or lateral position of the sac but also on the relationship of the diverticulum to the cricopharyngeus muscle. Diverticula may or may not be symptomatic, which is usually based on the size of the diverticulum. The presence of a diverticulum may cause halitosis and dysphagia. Food

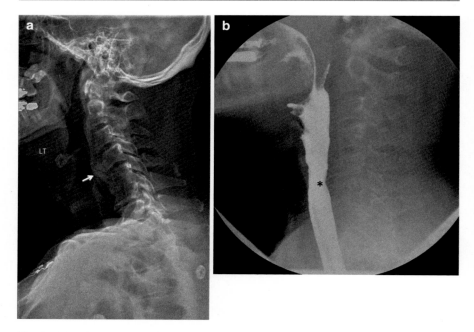

Fig. 6.13 Extrinsic compression by cervical osteophyte. (**a**) Large anterior marginal osteophytes at C4-C6 (*arrow*). (**b**) Cervical vertebral osteophytes in a different patient indenting the barium column during a single-contrast esophagram (*asterisk*)

entrapment within the diverticulum and esophageal dysmotility on account of the diverticulum or delayed reflux of food or liquid from the sac may all contribute to the development of symptoms. A mid-esophageal diverticulum may be formed by mediastinal adhesions and is a traction diverticulum (Fig. 6.17). It is formed due to extrinsic traction occurring as a result of fibrosis and scarring adjacent to the esophageal wall. An epiphrenic diverticulum is a distal esophageal diverticulum along the lateral esophageal wall and is usually a pulsion diverticulum, occurring as a result of asymmetric pressure along the esophageal wall (Fig. 6.18). The epiphrenic diverticulum is often associated with a hiatal hernia.

Esophagitis caused by acid reflux is a fairly common condition and may be seen in patients across a wide range of age groups. In addition to heartburn, reflux esophagitis may often present with dysphagia. Benign strictures of the esophagus [8, 9] may form as an end result of healing following reflux esophagitis (Fig. 6.11), candidiasis, or CMV infection of the esophagus in immunocompromised patients or following lye ingestion. Post-radiation therapy strictures are similar in appearance but the fibrosis may make them fixed and less distensible (Fig. 6.19). Assessment of malignant strictures includes at first the detection and then the differentiation from a benign stricture, followed by assessment of the location and extent of involvement [8, 9]. Achalasia is a neuromuscular disorder characterized by incomplete relaxation of the lower esophageal sphincter (LES) and the loss of primary peristaltic

Fig. 6.14 Ectatic aortic knob (*solid arrow*) causes mild narrowing of the cervical esophagus due to an extrinsic compression effect

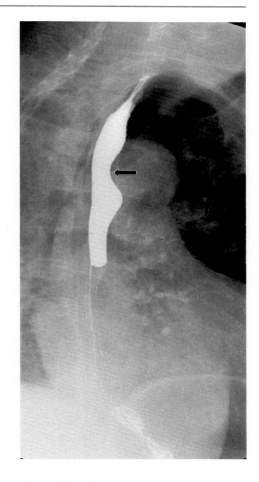

activity in the distal esophagus. This results in distention of most of the esophagus and a bird beak appearance of the distal esophagus [3] (Fig. 6.3a, b). When a column of barium is created during the esophagram, the increased pressure from the head of the column results in opening of the LES and passage of barium through the opened sphincter. This finding helps distinguish a fixed small segment distal esophageal stricture from achalasia. Achalasia may be primary, which is due to loss of ganglion cells in the myenteric plexus, or secondary, which may be due to esophageal carcinoma or a rare parasitic disease known as Chagas disease. Radiological findings are useful in distinguishing between these two types of the condition [10]. In primary achalasia, the narrowed segment averages 1.9 cm (range of 0.7–3.5 cm) and the dilated segment of the esophagus has a mean diameter of 6–2 cm (range of 4–10 cm.) In secondary achalasia, the narrowed segment is longer, averaging 4.1 cm (range of 3.5–6 cm), and the dilated pre-stricture esophageal segment has a diameter of 4 cm. or less. Esophageal carcinoma results in a slowly progressive dysphagia accompanied by constitutional symptoms of weakness and weight loss and may at

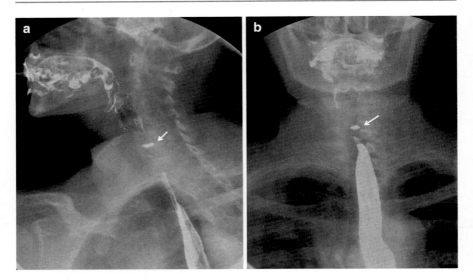

Fig. 6.15 Zenker's diverticulum. An outpouching (*arrow*) of the posterior esophageal wall is seen in the lateral projection (**a**) and in the frontal projection (**b**)

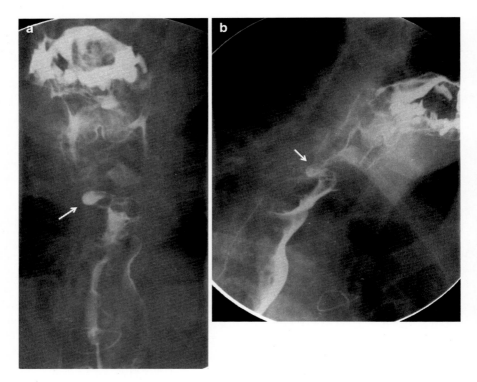

Fig. 6.16 Killian diverticulum (*arrow*) is an outpouching from the anterolateral wall of the cervical esophagus seen in the frontal projection (**a**) and with the patient in a LPO position (**b**)

Fig. 6.17 Traction diverticulum. This is a mid-esophageal diverticulum caused by traction from adjacent mediastinal fibrosis

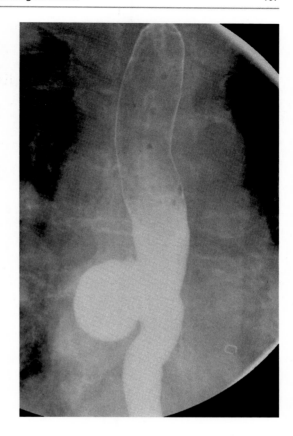

times be associated with the symptom of vomiting. Radiographically, this may manifest as secondary achalasia as detailed above or by the presence as an irregular, asymmetric stricture which may extend to the gastric cardia (Figs. 6.20 and 6.21). A hiatal hernia may result in a sensation of dysphagia (Fig. 6.22). A paraesophageal hernia can likewise cause dysphagia. In a paraesophageal hernia, the gastroesophageal junction remains in place at the diaphragmatic hiatus and a portion of the stomach herniates alongside the distal esophagus (Fig. 6.23a, b). The sensation of dysphagia may be caused by the delayed transit of the barium and pooling within the herniated portion of the stomach or due to alteration of esophageal peristaltic activity with tertiary contractions and resultant delay in bolus propulsion . Dysphagia in the setting of a hiatal hernia may also occur due to partial obstruction at the diaphragmatic hiatus or due to gastroesophageal reflux. A large hiatal hernia may result in an organoaxial volvulus [11] (Fig. 6.24). Due to the laxity of the gastric ligaments and the surrounding peritoneal reflections, the stomach may rotate with the greater curvature of the stomach ending up superior to the lesser curvature [11]. This has the potential to result in obstruction. Another not so uncommon cause of dysphagia is a foreign body lodged within the esophagus. In children, this may be an inadvertently swallowed foreign object or a part from a toy that may have come loose. In

Fig. 6.18 Epiphrenic
diverticulum. An outpouching
is seen arising from the left
lateral wall of the distal
esophagus (*arrow*), which is
caused by asymmetric
pressure along the wall of the
esophagus

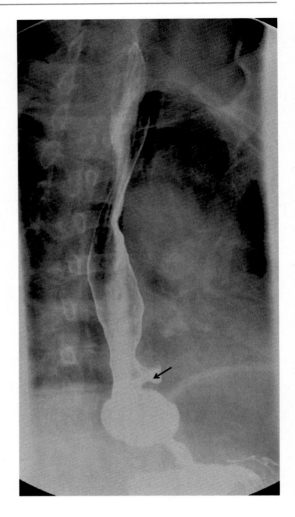

adults more often than not, the foreign body is a large piece of meat or other food
bolus which is incompletely chewed (Fig. 6.25). In the elderly, a part of a denture
may come loose and be swallowed during a meal. The onset of symptoms is usually
sudden in these cases, and the patient history is generally very helpful.

CT Scan

A CT scan of the neck, chest, or both may be obtained as an initial or secondary
imaging study in the assessment of dysphagia. The CT scan may be used to assess
the nature of a process that is seen to cause extrinsic compression on the pharynx or
esophagus, to evaluate the extraluminal extent of a disease process, and also for
staging a malignant neoplasm.

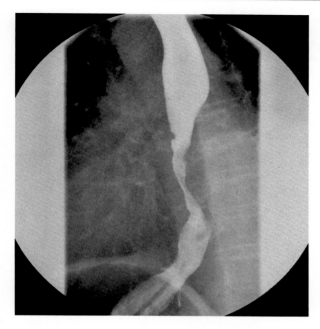

Fig. 6.19 Post-radiation stricture. Long segment stricture in the mid to distal esophagus due to radiation-related fibrosis in a patient with esophageal carcinoma

Procedure [12]

A multidetector scanner is utilized with postprocessing capability for multiplanar reconstruction after the initial axial data has been acquired. The patient is positioned supine with the neck slightly extended so as to exclude the orbits while scanning the neck. The gantry is angled parallel to the hard palate (Fig. 6.26). The patient receives a bolus of nonionic iodinated contrast intravenously via a peripheral vein that has been accessed at the start of the examination. Care is taken to flush out any air from the tubing that connects a power injector (Fig. 6.26) via the venous access line. Helical, axial images are obtained at a slice thickness of 3 mm. These are later reconstructed in the sagittal and coronal planes and made available for interpretation by the radiologist on a PACS system.

When imaging the chest, the patient is similarly positioned supine but with their arms raised above the head so as to prevent streak artifact across the chest. Intravenous contrast is administered by a power injector via a peripheral IV access line and helical axial images are obtained at a slice thickness of 5 mm; then reconstruction of the coronal and sagittal or sagittal oblique planes is deemed appropriate, on a case by case basis.

The CT scan provides excellent anatomic detail for diagnosis and treatment planning in patients with dysphagia.

Figure 6.27a–c demonstrate the normal anatomy of the neck. Various conditions may result in the symptom of dysphagia in the neck. A very commonly encountered condition, acute tonsillitis may cause dysphagia and odynophagia, or painful

Fig. 6.20 Distal esophageal
carcinoma. Irregularity along
the wall of the esophagus and
filling defects (*arrows*) in the
barium column caused by the
presence of a distal
esophageal malignancy

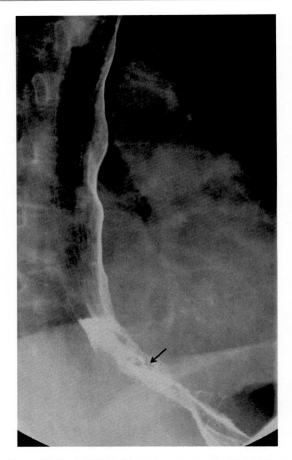

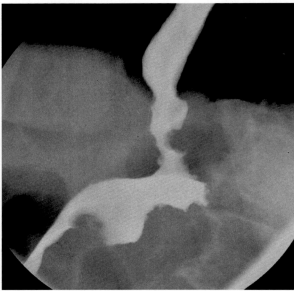

Fig. 6.21 Esophageal
carcinoma with extension to
the fundus and body of the
stomach. Irregularity along
the walls of the distal
esophagus and the proximal
stomach shows the extent of
the malignancy

Fig. 6.22 Hiatal hernia.
The fundus and a portion of
the body of the stomach have
herniated through the
diaphragmatic hiatus
(*arrows*)

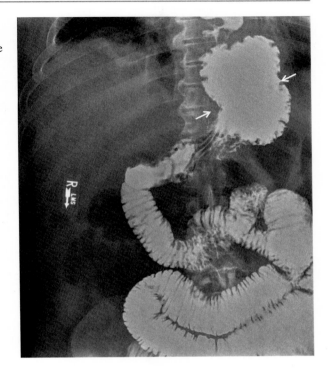

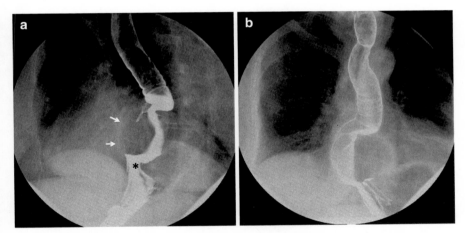

Fig. 6.23 Paraesophageal hernia. (**a**) A gas-filled portion of the stomach (*arrows*) has herniated
alongside the distal esophagus with the gastroesophageal junction positioned at the diaphragmatic
hiatus (*asterisk*). (**b**) Tertiary contractions are seen in the esophagus of the same patient with a
paraesophageal hernia

Fig. 6.24 Organoaxial
volvulus. The herniated
stomach has twisted along
its long axis resulting in the
greater curvature to the right
and superior to the lesser
curvature

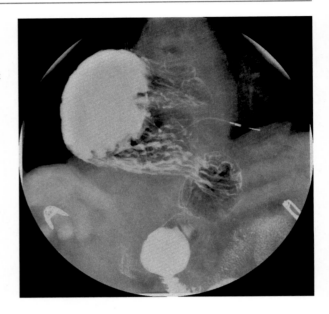

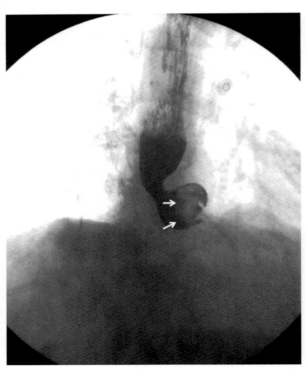

Fig. 6.25 Foreign body in
the esophagus. A filling
defect is seen in the distal
esophagus (*arrows*). A piece
of incompletely chewed
meat was retrieved at
endoscopy

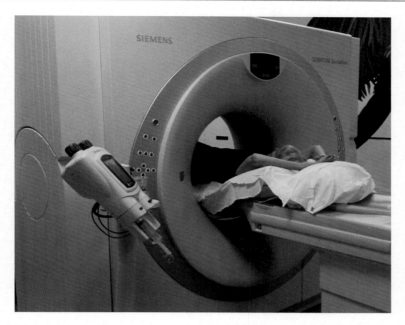

Fig. 6.26 Patient in the CT scanner, positioned with arms raised above the head for a CT scan of the chest. When obtaining a CT scan of the neck, the arms are placed beside the body. The power injector is in the foreground, adjacent to the gantry of the CT scanner

swallowing (Fig. 6.28). Although tonsillitis can be easily diagnosed clinically, the presence of a complication such as a peritonsillar abscess (Fig. 6.29a, b) may be detected or confirmed by CT in patients where the expected recovery does not occur in spite of antibiotic treatment or when suspected clinically in patients presenting later in the course of the infection. Confirmation with a neck CT allows for the appropriate surgical management. A retropharyngeal abscess (Fig. 6.30) may occur due to spread of infection to the retropharyngeal space from the peritonsillar or parapharyngeal region or from the pharynx itself. At times infection may spread from the vertebrae to the prevertebral and the retropharyngeal space and would result in dysphagia and odynophagia. Benign lesions such as a ranula or thyroglossal duct cyst may be diagnosed with confidence both by CT and MRI. A thyroglossal cyst is congenital and arises from the thyroglossal duct remnant, presenting in childhood or adolescence. A ranula is an acquired cystic lesion that occurs in the floor of the mouth due to obstruction of a sublingual salivary gland duct or the duct of a minor salivary gland in the sublingual region [13]. This may be a simple ranula which is confined to the sublingual space or a plunging ranula, which extends inferior to the mylohyoid muscle (Fig. 6.31). In the case of a laryngocele, it is possible to differentiate an internal laryngocele from a mixed internal and external

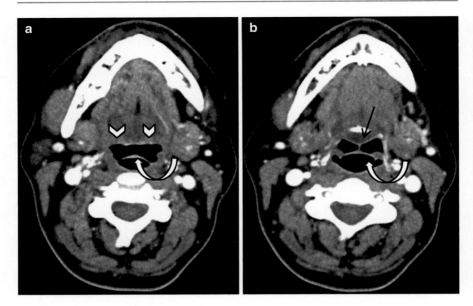

Fig. 6.27 Cross-sectional anatomy of the neck on CT scan images obtained from superior to inferior. The *arrowheads* in (**a**) show the tongue base. The free edge and base of the epiglottis are depicted by the *curved arrows* (**a**, **b**). The glossoepiglottic fold (*black arrow* in **b**) connects the tongue base to the base of the epiglottis and divides the pocket into two valecullae. The aryepiglottic folds, one on each side (*curved arrow* in **c**), separate the airway from the pyriform sinus which is the path taken by swallowed liquids and solid foods. The anterior commissure (*straight arrow* in **d**) is the apex at which the two vocal cords (*curved arrow* in **d**) come together. This is an important landmark when determining the type and extent of surgery for laryngeal carcinoma. The trachea (*T*) in image (**e**) maintains its shape and patency due to the presence of incomplete tracheal cartilaginous rings which are deficient posteriorly so as to allow for distensibility of the posteriorly positioned cervical esophagus. The thyroid gland (*white arrow* in **e**) drapes the trachea

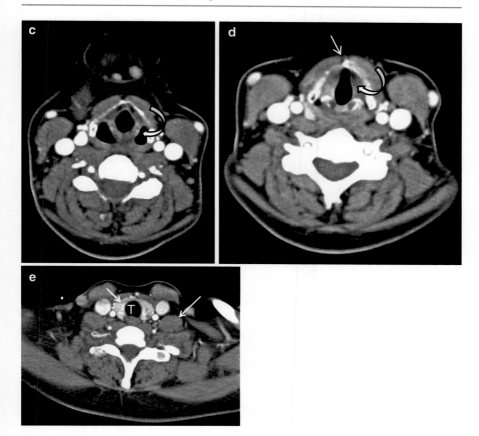

Fig. 6.27 (continued)

Fig. 6.28 Bilateral
tonsillitis. Bilateral
hypertrophied tonsils (*T*)
result in significant crowding
of the oropharyngeal space

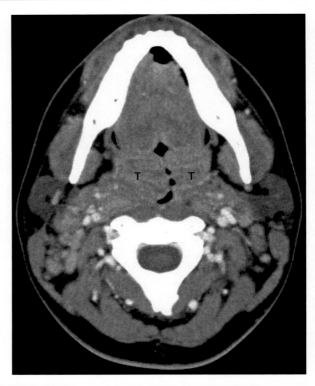

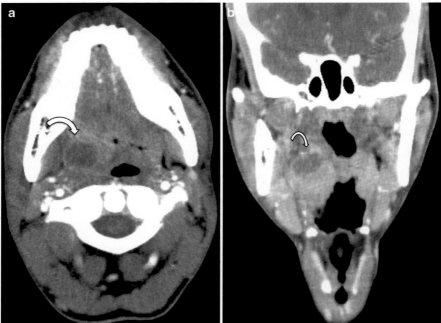

Fig. 6.29 Peritonsillar abscess. A contained fluid collection (*curved arrow*) is seen in the right peritonsillar space in the axial (**a**) and coronal reconstructed (**b**) images at the level of the oropharynx

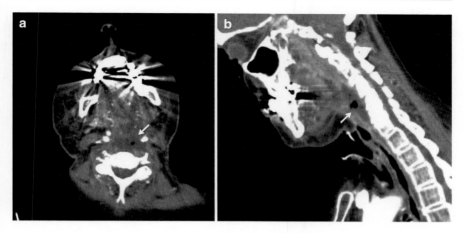

Fig. 6.30 Retropharyngeal abscess. An air-fluid collection (*arrow*) is seen in the retropharyngeal space on the axial (**a**) and sagittal reconstructed (**b**) CT images of the neck

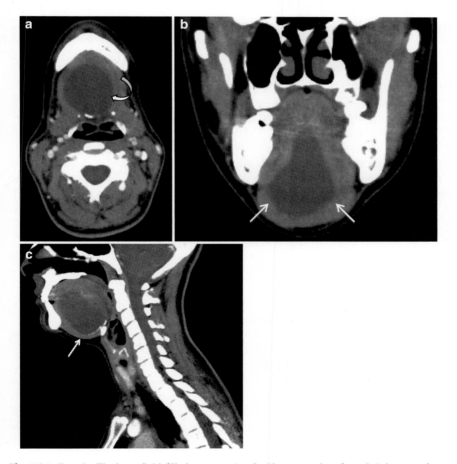

Fig. 6.31 Ranula. The large fluid-filled structure (marked by *arrows* in **a**, **b**, and **c**) denotes a large plunging ranula extending inferior to the mylohyoid muscle

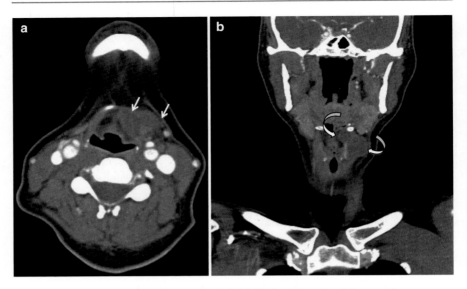

Fig. 6.32 Mixed laryngocele. (**a**) The bilobed fluid-filled structure (*straight arrows*) represents a mixed laryngocele seen in the axial plane. (**b**) Coronal reconstructed image (*curved arrows*) shows the two components of the mixed laryngocele

laryngocele (Fig. 6.32). A laryngocele is a cystic dilatation of the laryngeal saccule [14]. This may be congenital or acquired. Increased intraglottic pressure caused by excessive coughing, playing a wind instrument, or glass blowing can result in the formation of a laryngocele. Large laryngoceles can cause dysphagia due to mass effect on the pharynx. Other possible symptoms include stridor, hoarseness, snoring, and a neck mass. Laryngoceles may be internal (extending medially into the airway), external (extending laterally into the soft tissues of the neck through the thyrohyoid membrane), or mixed, i.e., combined internal and external [14, 15]. A laryngocele may be symptomatic due to its size and location, may be complicated by infection, and, although rare, can be associated with laryngeal carcinoma. It is for these reasons that a laryngocele needs to be appropriately evaluated with a CT scan or an MRI of the neck. A large hiatal hernia with a resultant organoaxial volvulus may come to light when a CT scan of the chest is obtained for chest pain or retrosternal discomfort (Fig. 6.33).

A head and neck malignancy is evaluated by CT for assessment of the extent of involvement and staging and for appropriate treatment planning [16] (Figs. 6.34 and 6.35). An assessment of response to treatment may be made utilizing the modalities of CT or PET-CT. An annual surveillance is generally done with a neck CT.

Mediastinal lesions can result in low dysphagia. These conditions are best evaluated with a chest CT. Mediastinal lesions may be responsible for dysphagia by causing extrinsic mass effect or by causing internal obstruction to the passage of a bolus. A thyroid goiter with mediastinal extension may cause extrinsic mass effect and at times a shift of the trachea away from the side of the goiter (Fig. 6.36). Bulky

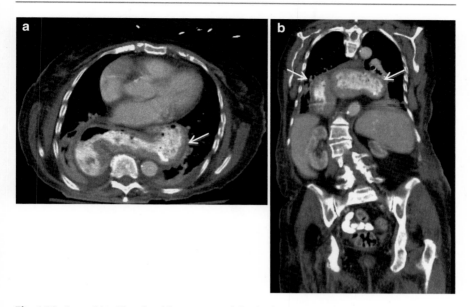

Fig. 6.33 Large hiatal hernia with an organoaxial volvulus. (**a**) An axial CT image shows a large hiatal hernia with most of the stomach (*arrows*) in an intrathoracic location. (**b**) The coronal reconstructed image shows to better advantage the organoaxial volvulus, with the greater curvature of the stomach positioned superiorly (*arrows*)

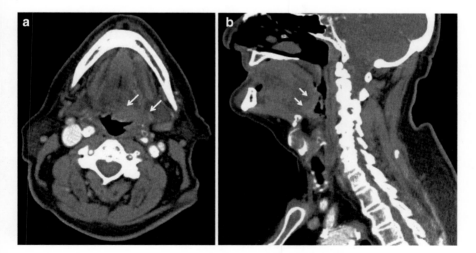

Fig. 6.34 Tongue base carcinoma. (**a**) There is an irregular, enhancing mass (*arrows*) seen arising from the left tongue base, extending across the midline and also extending to the left lateral pharyngeal wall. This is seen in the axial plane. (**b**) The sagittal reconstructed image shows the craniocaudal extent of the mass

Fig. 6.35 An irregular, enhancing soft-tissue mass is seen (*arrows*) involving the epiglottis and the left valecula. This represents a supraglottic malignancy

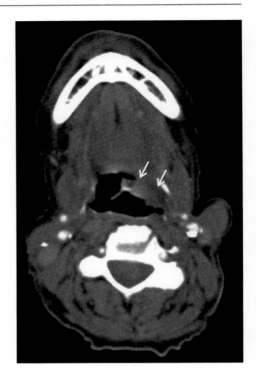

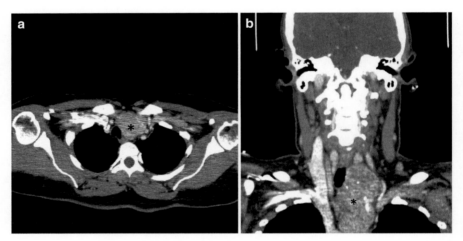

Fig. 6.36 (**a**) An axial CT image shows an enlarged thyroid gland, or goiter (*asterisk*). (**b**) The same is also seen in a reconstructed image in the coronal plane where the goiter is seen to have intrathoracic extension. Images obtained through the chest subsequently (not shown here) were able to reveal the entire mediastinal extent of the goiter

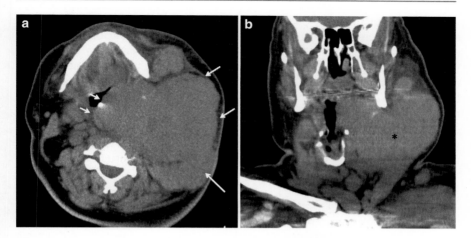

Fig. 6.37 Non-Hodgkin's lymphoma. (**a**) A large, bulky, lobular mass (*arrows*) is present in the left side of the neck causing significant mass effect and resultant airway and oropharyngeal compromise. (**b**) Coronal reconstructed image shows the cranio-caudal and medial extent of the tumor (*asterisk*)

mediastinal lymphadenopathy such as that which occurs in chronic granulomatous disease, lymphoma, or lymph node metastases can at times cause dysphagia on account of mass effect and extrinsic compression (Fig. 6.37). Malignant neoplasms of the mucosa or wall of the pharyngo-esophageal tract can result in gradual onset of dysphagia with progression of symptoms. Other coexisting local and systemic symptoms may be present that raise clinical suspicion of the disease process. A malignant neoplasm involving anywhere from the oral cavity to the esophagus and gastroesophageal junction may result in dysphagia. A CT scan of the neck and chest is a useful test to assess the extent of involvement by the primary tumor and also to evaluate for metastases [15]. This allows for staging of the malignancy and provides information for putting together the treatment plan best suited to that patient.

MRI

An MRI of the neck and when need of the face allows for multiplanar assessment of the area of concern. Location of the lesion and the signal characteristics help the radiologist in rendering a useful differential diagnosis or in certain classic cases may afford the only diagnosis. The multiplanar capability of MRI is very useful in evaluating the true extent of the disease process. In cases of malignancy, this is important for accurate staging and treatment planning. In benign lesions, it affords valuable information to the surgeon regarding the involvement of adjoining structures, tissue planes, and estimated surgical time.

Patient preparation: The patient answers a relevant MRI safety questionnaire. Provided that there are no contraindications such as an intracranial metallic aneurysm clip, a cardiac pacemaker, low effective GFR if receiving intravenous gadolinium contrast, or contrast allergy, the patient may proceed to the MRI scanner. At our facilities, there is availability to test the BUN and creatinine on site, should there be any doubt of renal insufficiency. Although allergy to MRI contrast material is rare, it has been known to occur and so this is always asked about. Certain metallic devices are MRI compatible and it is prudent that the patient brings along any relevant information regarding implanted devices. The patient needs to be NPO for 4 h prior to the procedure when intravenous contrast is to be administered.

Procedure

The patient is positioned supine on the MRI table in the bore of the magnet. A 1.5 or 3 T magnet may be used depending on availability. The patient gets to choose the music he/she would like to listen to during the exam. Some patients prefer to wear occlusive earbuds. Either one helps reduce the discomfort of the loud sound that is produced by the RF pulse during the examination. A dedicated neck coil is placed and the patient prepared for scanning. If intravenous contrast is being used, an IV line is secured and the power injector attached. Precontrast and post-contrast sequences are obtained in the axial, coronal, and sagittal planes.

An MRI of the neck is a useful study for detecting small lesions that may not have been evident on endoscopic evaluation or on a CT examination. The high grayscale contrast allows for better definition of tissue planes surrounding a lesion. The multiplanar capability is very useful for assessing the extent of a disease process.

Benign lesions such as a ranula or thyroglossal duct cyst may be diagnosed with confidence both by CT and MRI. The characteristics of a ranula have been described in detail previously. A plunging ranula extends inferior to the mylohyoid muscle (Fig. 6.38) and appears T1 dark and T2 bright with no contrast enhancement or mild wall enhancement if there is mild inflammation or if the lesion has been previously infected. Lesions within the soft tissues of the neck may can at times result in vague discomfort during swallowing or present as neck swellings. The location and signal characteristics of such a lesion may afford a very good differential diagnosis aiding in further management and in instances of classic presentation allow the radiologist to pinpoint the diagnosis itself as in the case of a schwannoma (Fig. 6.39). Evaluation of local invasion and metastasis to cervical lymph nodes can be made with accuracy.

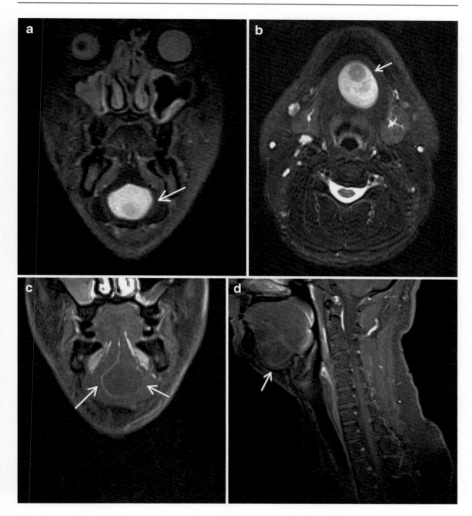

Fig. 6.38 Ranula MRI images. (**a**) Coronal T2 image shows a T2 bright circumscribed lesion in the submental space (*arrow*). (**b**) Axial T2 image showing the same lesion (*arrow*). (**c**) Coronal fat-sat post-contrast T1 image shows a T1 dark lesion with peripheral enhancement but no internal enhancement (*arrow*). (**d**) Sagittal fat-sat post-contrast T1 image showing the same lesion (*arrow*)

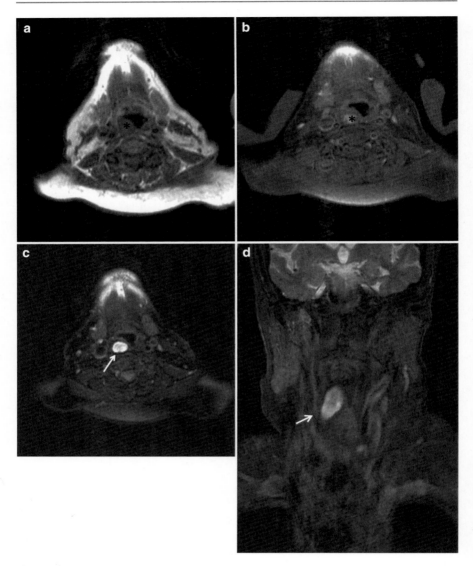

Fig. 6.39 MRI images of a parapharyngeal mass – schwannoma. (**a**) T1 axial image shows a T1 isointense parapharyngeal tumor (*black asterisk*). (**b**) T2 fat-sat axial image shows an hyperintense lesion (*black asterisk*) in the right parapharyngeal space. (**c**) T1 fat-sat post-contrast axial image shows an intensely enhancing right parapharyngeal mass (*arrow*). (**d**) T1 fat-sat post-contrast coronal image shows the same enhancing right parapharyngeal mass (*arrow*) in a different plane

Conclusion

Radiological testing has advanced in the past several years and affords an excellent diagnostic evaluation in patients with dysphagia. The different modalities, namely, fluoroscopic evaluation, CT scan, and MRI, are useful individually or in combination to make an accurate diagnosis.

References

1. Daniels SK, Ballo LA, et al. Clinical predictors of dysphagia and aspiration risk: outcome measures in acute stroke patients. Arch Phys Med Rehabil. 2000;81(8):1030–3.
2. Rubesin SE, Levine MS. Killian-Jamieson diverticula: radiographic findings in 16 patients. AJR Am J Roentgenol. 2001;177:85–9.
3. Woodfield CA, Levine MS, et al. Diagnosis of primary versus secondary achalasia: reassessment of clinical and radiographic criteria. AJR Am J Roentgenol. 2000;175:727–31.
4. Muller M, Goekel I, Hedwig P, et al. Is the Schatzki ring a unique esophageal entity? World J Gastroenterol. 2011;17(23):2838–93.
5. Practice Guidelines and Technical Standards Handbook – American College of Radiology. Revised 2013. Reston, VA. www.acr.org
6. Eisenberg RL. Gastrointestinal radiology: a pattern approach. 4th ed. Philadelphia: Lippincott-Raven Publishers; 1996.
7. Prabhakar A, Levine MS, et al. Relationship between diffuse esophageal spasm and lower esophageal sphincter dysfunction on barium studies and manometry in 14 patients. Am J Roentgenol. 2004;183:409–13.
8. Karasick S, Leu-Toaff AS. Esophageal strictures: findings on barium radiographs. AJR Am J Roentgenol. 1995;165:561–5.
9. Luedtke PA, Levine MS, Rubesin SE, et al. Radiographic diagnosis of benign esophageal strictures: a pattern approach. Radiographics. 2003;23(4):897–909.
10. Gupta S, Levine MS, Rubesin SE, et al. Usefulness of barium studies for differentiating benign and malignant strictures of the esophagus. AJR Am J Roentgenol. 2003;180:737–44.
11. Peterson CM, Anderson JS, et al. Volvulus of the gastrointestinal tract: appearances at multi-modality imaging. Radiographics. 2009;29:1281–93.
12. ACR-ASNR-SPR Practice Guidelines for the performance of CT of the extracranial head and neck.pdf Revised 2011. http://www.asnr.org/sites/default/files/guidelines/CT_Head_Neck.pdf
13. Coit WE, Harnsberger HR, Osborn AG, et al. Ranulas and their mimics: CT evaluation. Radiology. 1987;163(1):211–6.
14. Glazer HS, Mauro MA, Aronberg DJ, et al. Computed tomography of laryngoceles. AJR Am J Roentgenol. 1983;140:549–52.
15. Lancella A, Abbate G, Dosdegan R. Mixed laryngocele: a case report and review of literature. Acta Otorhinolaryngol Ital. 2007;27(5):255–7.
16. Gilbert K, Dalley RW, Maronian N, Anzai Y. Staging of laryngeal cancer using 64-channel multidetector row CT: comparison of standard neck CT with dedicated breath maneuver laryngeal CT. AJNR Am J Neuroradiol. 2010;31:251–6.

Neurogenic Dysphagia

7

Charu Sankhla and Kirti Bharambe

The understanding of normal physiology and pathophysiology of eating and swallowing disorders is essential for evaluating and managing disorders of eating and swallowing and developing dysphagia rehabilitation programs. Eating and swallowing are complex activities including both volitional and reflexive activities involving more than 30 nerves and muscles [1].

Disturbances in the mouth, tongue, pharynx, or esophagus can impair swallowing [dysphagia][1]. It can involve mechanical, musculoskeletal, or neurogenic mechanisms. This chapter will focus on neuromuscular and neurogenic causes of dysphagia because the diseases in these categories are seen by the neurologist.

Commonly used models to describe the physiology of normal eating and swallowing are four-stage model for drinking and swallowing liquid and the process model for eating and swallowing solid food. The normal swallow in humans is a three-stage sequential model. The swallowing process is divided into oral, pharyngeal, and esophageal stages according to the location of the bolus [2, 3]. The oral stage is subdivided into oral preparatory and oral propulsive stages, which resulted in four-stage model. Studies on the four-stage model adequately describe biomechanism and bolus movement during voluntary swallows of liquids. However, this model lacked understanding of the bolus movement and the process of eating of solid food. Therefore, the process model of feeding was established to describe the mechanism of eating and swallowing of solid food [4, 5].

C. Sankhla (✉) • K. Bharambe
Neurology, P. D. Hinduja Hospital, Mahim, Mumbai, India
e-mail: charusankhla@gmail.com

© Springer India 2015
G. Mankekar (ed.), *Swallowing – Physiology, Disorders, Diagnosis and Therapy*,
DOI 10.1007/978-81-322-2419-8_7

Oral Preparatory Stage

After liquid is taken into the mouth from a cup or by a straw, the liquid bolus is held in the anterior part of the floor of the mouth or on the tongue surface against the hard palate surrounded by the upper dental arch (upper teeth). The soft palate seals oral cavity and tongue contact to prevent the liquid bolus leaking into the oropharynx before the swallow. There can be leakage of liquid into the pharynx if the seal is imperfect. The impairment of this mechanism occurs with aging.

Oral Propulsive Stage

During oral propulsive stage, the tongue tip rises, touching the alveolar ridge of the hard palate just behind the upper teeth, while the posterior tongue drops to open the back of the oral cavity. The tongue surface moves upward, gradually expanding the area of tongue-palate contact from anterior to posterior, squeezing the liquid bolus back along the palate and into the pharynx. When drinking liquids, the pharyngeal stage normally begins during oral propulsion.

Oral Stage in Eating Solid Food (Process Model of Feeding)

The four-stage sequential model was unable to explain normal eating in humans, especially food transport and bolus formation in the oropharynx [4–6].

When healthy subjects eat solid food, it is chewed and moistened. It passes through the fauces for bolus formation in the oropharynx (including the valleculae) several seconds prior to the pharyngeal stage of a swallow. Additional portions of food can pass into the oropharynx and accumulate there while food remains in the oral cavity and chewing continues. Eating and swallowing solid food is a continuous process unlike swallowing liquids and, hence, cannot be explained by four-stage model. There is an overlap in oral preparatory, propulsive, and pharyngeal stage of swallowing solids. Hence, process model based on studies in mammalian is adapted.

Stage I Transport

The ingested food is carried and placed in occlusal surface of lower teeth for processing.

Food Processing

In this stage, food particles are chewed to small size and softened by salivation until the food consistency is optimal for swallowing. Chewing continues until it is of optimal consistency for swallowing. Chewing is continuous process till it is ready for swallowing. The movements of jaw, tongue, cheek, soft palate, and hyoid bone are preferably coordinated.

Movements of the Jaw, Hyoid, and Tongue or Soft Palate Over Time

During this, there is an open passage between oral cavity and pharynx unlike closure of posterior oral cavity during drinking liquids [5, 7]. Movements of the jaw and tongue pump air into the nasal cavity through the pharynx, delivering the food's aroma to chemoreceptors in the nose [8–10].

The tongue movements are coordinated with jaw opening and closing in such a manner as to avoid tongue coordinated by suprahyoid and infrahyoid muscles. These muscles help to control the movements of the jaw and tongue as well [11, 12].

Stage II Transport

The masticated food is placed on the tongue surface and pushed back to the oropharynx. The basic mechanism of stage II transport is as described for the oral propulsive stage with a liquid bolus. (The anterior tongue surface first contacts the hard palate just behind the upper incisors. The area of tongue-palate contact gradually expands backward, squeezing the masticated food back along the palate to the oropharynx.) Stage II transport involves the tongue and does not require gravity [13, 14] and can be along with food processing cycles. The transported food accumulates on the pharyngeal surface of the tongue and in the valleculae. If food remains in the oral cavity, chewing continues and the bolus in the oropharynx is enlarged by subsequent stage II transport cycles. The duration of bolus aggregation in the oropharynx ranges from a fraction of a second to about 10 s in normal individuals eating solid food [5].

Pharyngeal Stage

Pharyngeal swallow occurs in seconds. During this phase, bolus is propelled to pharynx and to esophagus simultaneously closing larynx and trachea preventing food from entering the airway. As the soft palate elevates, the nasopharynx closes at the same time and prevents bolus regurgitation in the nasal cavity. The base of the tongue retracts, pushing the bolus against the pharyngeal walls. The pharyngeal constrictor muscles contract sequentially from the top to the bottom, squeezing the bolus downward. This reduces the volume of pharyngeal cavity.

Prevention of aspiration during swallowing is very essential in human beings. (There are several airway protective mechanisms preventing aspiration of the foreign materials to the trachea before or during swallowing.) During swallowing, vocal folds adduct to close the glottis (space between the vocal folds) and the arytenoids tilt forward to contact the epiglottic base prior to opening of the UES [15, 16]. Suprahyoid muscles and thyrohyoid muscle contract to pull hyoid and larynx upward and forward. (This displacement tucks the larynx under the base of the tongue. The epiglottis tilts backward to seal the laryngeal vestibule.)

Opening of the upper esophageal sphincter (UES) is essential for the bolus entry into the esophagus. The UES consists of the inferior pharyngeal constrictor muscles, cricopharyngeus muscle, and most proximal part of the esophagus. The UES is closed at rest by tonic muscle contraction [17, 18]. Three important factors contribute to the UES opening: (1) relaxation of the cricopharyngeus muscle; this relaxation normally precedes opening of the UES or arrival of the bolus; (2) contraction of the suprahyoid muscles and thyrohyoid muscles. These muscles pull the hyolaryngeal complex forward, opening the sphincter; and (3) the pressure of the descending bolus [19]. This pressure distends the UES, assisting its opening. The most important of these mechanisms is factor 2, the active opening process. This makes opening of the UES quite different from other sphincters (such as the external urethral sphincter which opens passively when it is pushed open by the descending fluid).

Esophageal Stage

The esophagus is a tubular structure from the lower part of the UES to the lower esophageal sphincter (LES). The lower esophageal sphincter is also tensioned at rest to prevent regurgitation from the stomach. It relaxes during a swallow and allows the bolus passage to the stomach. The cervical esophagus (upper one third) is mainly composed of striated muscle, but the thoracic esophagus (lower two thirds) is smooth muscle. Bolus transport in the thoracic esophagus is quite different from that of the pharynx, because it is true peristalsis regulated by the autonomic nervous system. Once the food bolus enters the esophagus passing the UES, a peristalsis wave carries the bolus down to the stomach through the LES. The peristaltic wave consists of two main parts, an initial wave of relaxation that accommodates the bolus, followed by a wave of contraction that propels it. Gravity assists peristalsis in upright position.

Bolus Location at Swallow Initiation in Normal Swallows

The position of the head of the bolus relative to the time of pharyngeal swallow onset is a measure of swallow elicitation. The point where the x-ray shadow of the ramus of the mandible crosses the pharyngeal surface of the tongue is commonly used as a marker for this measurement. At one time, it was believed that the pharyngeal swallow was normally triggered when the bolus head passes the fauces as seen on videofluoroscopy [3]. If the bolus head passed the lower border of the mandible more than 1 s before the swallow initiation, it was classified as delayed swallow initiation. Delayed swallow initiation is considered an important finding because the airway is open when the bolus approaches toward the larynx.

However, recent studies have revealed that pre-swallow bolus entry into the pharynx also occurs in healthy individuals drinking liquids [20–22]. Furthermore, as described above, during eating of solid food, chewed bolus is aggregated in the oropharynx or valleculae prior to swallowing. Bolus position at swallow initiation is now known to be quite variable in normal eating and swallowing. This is especially true when consuming a food that has both liquid and solid phases. Saitoh et al. [14] demonstrated that in healthy young adult eating a food that included soft solid and thin liquid components, the leading edge (liquid component) of the food often entered the hypopharynx before swallowing. As seen in, liquid enters the hypopharynx during chewing and approaches the laryngeal aditus at a time when the larynx remains open. The location of the bolus at swallow initiation is altered by sequential swallowing of liquid [20, 23–26]. The bolus head often reaches the valleculae before pharyngeal swallow initiation, especially when the larynx remains closed between swallows.

Coordination among Eating, Swallowing, and Breathing

Eating, swallowing, and breathing are tightly coordinated. Swallowing is dominant to respiration in normal individuals [27–29]. Breathing ceases briefly during swallowing, not only because of the physical closure of the airway by elevation of the soft palate and tilting of the epiglottis, but also of neural suppression of respiration in the brain stem [28]. When drinking a liquid bolus, swallowing usually starts during the expiratory phase of breathing. The respiratory pause continues for 0.5–1.5 s during swallowing, and respiration usually resumes with expiration [30–32]. This resumption is regarded as one of the mechanisms that prevent inhalation of food remaining in the pharynx after swallowing [33]. When performing sequential swallows while drinking from a cup, respiration can resume with inspiration [34].

Eating solid food also alters the respiratory rhythm. The rhythm is perturbed with onset of mastication. Respiratory cycle duration decreases during mastication, but with swallowing [29, 35, 36]. The "exhale-swallow-exhale" temporal relationship persists during eating. However, respiratory pauses are longer, often beginning substantially before swallow onset [10, 36, 37].

Causes of Neurogenic Dysphagia

Normal swallowing depends on the anatomical and functional integrity of numerous neural structures and extensive pathways in the central and peripheral nervous system. Lesions of the cerebral cortex, basal ganglia, brain stem, cerebellum, and lower cranial nerves may result in dysphagia. Degenerations of the myenteric ganglion cells in the esophagus, muscle diseases, and disorders of neuromuscular transmission, for example, myasthenia gravis and Eaton-Lambert syndrome, are other less common causes.

Cerebral Cortex

The stroke is the commonest cortical condition associated with dysphagia; one fourth to half cases of all strokes are associated with swallowing difficulty [38]. Dysphagia in these patients is usually associated with hemiplegia due to lesions of the brain stem or the involvement of one or both hemispheres. Rarely isolated dysphagia is presenting symptom of stroke. Dysphagia is seen in patients with lacunar infarcts in the periventricular white matter [39] and after discrete vascular brain stem lesions [40]. These patients may not have associated neurological deficit. The swallowing difficulty in acute stroke is usually transient lasting for 2 weeks in most.

The symptoms persist in about 8 % of patients for 6 months or more [41]. The occurrence of dysphagia in acute stroke does not appear to depend on the size or the site of the lesion. Right parietal strokes are associated with persistent dysphagia.

Basal Ganglia

Dysphagia is a common symptom in patients with Parkinson's disease particularly in the later stages of the disease. Occasionally, dysphagia may even be a presenting symptom of Parkinson's disease.

More than 80 % of patients with Parkinson's disease have mild dysphagia, and usually, patient's nutritional status is well maintained. However, in about 10 % of dysphagic Parkinsonian patients, the symptoms are severe, and this generally correlates with the severity and duration of the disease. Tremor and speech disturbances have been found to be the main predictors of dysphagia in these patients [42].

The swallowing difficulties seen in Parkinson's disease involve the oral phase (difficulties with lip closure and tongue movements) and the pharyngeal stage (complaints of food sticking in the throat). Dysphagia is due to abnormal bolus formation, multiple tongue elevations, delayed swallow reflex, and prolongation of the pharyngeal transit time with repetitive swallows to clear the throat as shown on videofluoroscopy. Drooling, which is commonly seen in patients with Parkinsonism, is not due to excessive salivation but is due to impaired swallowing due to bradykinesia of the oropharyngeal musculature. Other Parkinsonian syndromes, for example, progressive supranuclear palsy and multisystem atrophy, cause more severe symptoms.

Dysphagia is also common in spasmodic torticollis. Videofluoroscopy revealed impairment of swallowing in more than half the patients [43]. Interestingly, only two thirds of the study patients were symptomatic and were independent of patient's age or disease duration. The dysphagia may be due to dystonia of laryngeal and pharyngeal muscle involvement. The nomenclature now is cervical dystonia than spasmodic torticollis.

Cerebellum and Brain Stem

The oral phase is affected in cerebellum and brain stem lesions due to bulbar or pseudobulbar palsy; this leads to poor coordination of the oral and pharyngeal musculature resulting in poor lip seal, impaired initiation of the swallow reflex, poorly formed food bolus, and its propulsion to the pharynx.

Peripheral Nerves and Muscles

The rare causes of dysphagia are isolated peripheral nerve lesions and degeneration of autonomic ganglion cells in the lower two thirds of the esophagus (which results in achalasia). This causes stagnation of food and dilatation of esophagus due to abnormally reduced motility of the lower esophagus with tightening of the sphincter. The diagnosis is confirmed with endoscopy and studies of esophageal motility. Common symptom in addition includes halitosis.

Myasthenia gravis is a neuromuscular junction abnormality. Dysphagia is commonly associated with dysphonia and dysarthria. The weakness is often fluctuating and may not be evident at the time of examination. The swallowing is commonly affected in elderly myasthenics. The diagnosis of the underlying disorder can usually be confirmed with single-fiber electromyography.

Drugs and Dysphagia

Many drugs may precipitate or aggravate swallowing difficulties. This effect is usually dose dependent and is often reversible with discontinuation of the drug. Sometimes, reduction of the drug dose is sufficient. The mechanisms implicated in drug-induced dysphagia include reduced level of consciousness (sedatives and hypnotics) causing interference with the oropharyngeal phase of swallowing or as a direct effect on brain stem neurons or blocking of acetylcholine release at the neuromuscular junction. Some drugs mediate their effect on swallowing by more than one mechanism.

Initiation of swallowing reflex is delayed by neuroleptics [dopamine-blocking agents] in absence of extrapyramidal features. Dopaminergic drugs can cause orofacial dyskinesia which interferes with the preparation of the food bolus and its delivery to the pharynx. Anticholinergic drugs cause dryness of mouth with impaired bolus formation with dysphagia. The benzodiazepines can cause impaired level of consciousness and suppress brain stem neurons that regulate swallowing [44, 45].

Botulinum toxin type A causes dysphagia due to inhibition of neural transmission at the neuromuscular junction. It is the drug of choice for the treatment of cervical dystonia and may cause dysphagia in 10–28 % of these patients. This adverse effect is usually mild and transient, lasting 10–14 days. Clinical observations suggest that the incidence of dysphagia is increased when a large dose of the drug is injected. It should also be noted that cervical dystonia may also be associated with dysphagia.

Clinical Manifestations of Dysphagia and Pulmonary Aspiration

Patients with mild to moderate difficulty in swallowing may not be aware of the swallowing difficulty, and weight loss may be the only symptom. Patients tend to drool in sitting position and may cough in the night due to silent aspiration.

Swallowing assessment would include inspection of oral cavity and small quantity trial swallows. Pooling of saliva in the oral cavity would indicate difficulty in swallowing liquids. Different consistencies of food and liquids should be tried. Watch for coughing and choking while eating; they are obvious signs. Change in the voice and observation of breathing pattern may be early signs. Making patient swallow water in upright position and observing their speed of swallowing are a quick bedside method of assessing swallowing [46]. The speed of swallowing is reduced to 10 ml/s and may indicate neurogenic dysphagia. Regular and frequent monitoring of swallowing is possible by this simple method. The other methods to assess swallowing include videofluoroscopy, fiber-optic nasoendoscopy, and pulse oximetry [47]. Videofluoroscopy allows direct visualization of oral preparatory phase, reflex initiation of swallowing, and actual passage of bolus in the pharyngeal phase, and direct aspiration in the respiratory tract can be seen. The disadvantages of this test include its unsuitability for repeated assessments. Fiber-optic endoscopy involves placing endoscope just above the soft palate and observing pharyngeal pooling before and after swallowing.

Patients with neurogenic dysphagia find fluids more difficult to swallow than solids. A solid food bolus is more likely to trigger a swallow reflex than liquid. Dysphagia resulting from brain stem lesions or confluent periventricular infarction may affect predominantly the volitional initiation of swallowing. Reflex swallowing is normal in such patients. Swallowing is associated with severe emotional distress, and patient complains of a lump in the throat. These patients have a normal bolus transit time and do not complain of difficulties with eating or drinking.

Complications of Dysphagia

The most dreaded complication of difficulty in swallowing is pulmonary aspiration. In addition, patient's caloric intake may be affected resulting in loss of weight. Reduced liquid intake may result in dehydration.

Pulmonary aspiration is defined as passage of food or fluid into the airways below the true vocal cords. Silent aspiration may go undetected unless clinician has high index of suspicion and may only be detected on pulse oximetry. One third of patients with difficulty in swallowing tend to aspirate their food or liquids in their airway, and 40 % of these patients have silent aspiration. Silent aspiration does not trigger coughing or cause distress. The patients often do not complain of swallowing difficulties. Weak cough may be one of the symptoms of early silent aspiration.

Management

Multidisciplinary approach is essential for management of neurogenic dysphagia. The team includes speech and language therapist, a dietician, a nurse, and a physician.

The causes of dysphagia are oral problems which result in poor food bolus formation. Poorly fitted dentures should be corrected, and mouth ulcers and candida infection should be treated. Avoid feeding patients when distracted particularly while watching television or talking. This increases the risk of aspiration. The suction should be carried out to remove saliva. Parkinson's patients experience on/off phenomenon. The swallowing may be normal in "on" state and impaired remarkably in "off" state.

Aspiration of saliva makes it necessary to do frequent suctioning of oral cavity. In dysphagic patients who have a tracheostomy, occlusion of the stoma with a speech valve during swallowing reduces the risk of pulmonary aspiration presumably by normalizing the pressure in the upper airways. Posture during swallowing is very important. For example, "chin tuck" decreases the pharyngeal transit time of the food bolus, whereas "chin up" has the opposite effect. Head tilt to one side to maximize the effect of gravity on the unaffected side of pharynx is also a useful strategy on some occasions.

It has been shown that patients with weak tongue movements and those with poor pharyngeal clearance of the food bolus benefit from the use of gravity and posture to facilitate safe swallowing. Lying down on one side (at 45° from flat) may be associated with less risk of aspiration than feeding in the upright position [48, 49].

Sedative and other drugs that reduce the patient's level of consciousness should be discontinued. In patients with Parkinson's disease, drug-induced dyskinesia may aggravate dysphagia, and the successful management of this complication usually improves swallowing. Sometimes, it is sufficient to avoid feeding during periods of peak-dose dyskinesia. Drooling in Parkinsonian patients is primarily due to swallowing difficulties rather than the excessive production of saliva. Anticholinergic drugs can aggravate dysphagia by increasing the viscosity of oral secretions. Viscid secretions interfere with bolus preparation and predispose to the formation of a mucous plug. Hence, these drugs are avoided in Parkinson patients with dysphagia. Benzodiazepines should be avoided in dysphagic patients, and anticonvulsants should be taken as a single dose at bedtime if possible.

Dietary Modification

Avoidance of dry and sticky food and eating food with uniform consistency and the use of starch-based fluid thickeners are also an important management strategy. Tube feeding is usually required in only a minority of patients.

Patients with neurogenic dysphagia experience more difficulties with fluids than with solid food. This is probably due to the difficulty in controlling a thin bolus and a delay or absence of triggering the swallow reflex. The rationale for the use of fluid thickeners is that by increasing the viscosity of ingested fluids, the resistance to flow of the bolus is increased. In addition, the duration of cricopharyngeal opening and the oropharyngeal transit time are increased. However, the optimal viscosity of fluids that ensures safe swallowing in patients with neurogenic dysphagia has not been established. In practice, the required fluid thickness is judged subjectively and recorded using descriptive terms such as syrup or yogurt consistency. This has the disadvantage that fluids with low viscosity may be served and result in pulmonary aspiration. Thick fluids are usually unpalatable and are often disliked by patients. A viscometer may be utilized to prepare correct thickness and has been shown to improve the dietary management in these cases [50].

Tube Feeding

Patients who are at risk of pulmonary aspiration if fed orally should be tube fed. Increased transit time of the food bolus on videofluoroscopy [51] may be indication for tube feeding. In some cases, easy fatigability makes swallowing unsafe; tube feeding can be used to supplement the daily oral intake. The patients are able to take their favorite foods orally, and the rest of the calorie requirements will be given through the tube.

The use of a gastrostomy tube is preferred to nasoesophageal intubation, especially in prolonged dysphagia. Nasogastric tube feeding is poorly tolerated. Patient may get irritable or agitated. Patients commonly extubate themselves; the volume of feeds delivered is inadequate. Patients fed using a nasogastric tube received less feeds as compared to those fed with a gastrostomy tube [52]; nasogastric tube uses fine-bore tubes, which are more likely to dislodge, kink, or block. They also deliver feeds at a relatively slow rate.

Some patients with neurological disease develop gastrointestinal ileus, and in these patients, enteral nutrition could be established with the intrajejunal administration of low-residue solutions.

Prolonged nasogastric tube feeding often results in nasopharyngitis, esophagitis, esophageal strictures, epistaxis, pneumothorax, and nasopharyngeal edema with associated otitis media. Furthermore, nasogastric tube feeding does not fully protect against aspiration, and the association between nasogastric tube feeding and this complication is well documented. Forty-three percent of dysphagic patients aspirated in the first 2 weeks after nasogastric tube feeding was started Ciocon et al. [53]. Elevation of the head of the bed during and for 1–2 h after feeding reduces the risk of aspiration in these patients.

Most clinicians would consider gastrostomy tube feeding in stroke patients if there are no signs of recovery of swallowing after the first week. In patients with motor neuron disease, the option of percutaneous endoscopic gastrostomy (PEG) tube feeding should be offered early after the onset of dysphagia to supplement the oral intake and help maintain the muscle mass. Insertion of the feeding tube through a PEG, rather than a surgical gastrostomy, is a relatively simple, safe, and cost-effective technique. PEG tube feeding is effective and is usually acceptable to patients and their caretakers. Transient, self-limiting abdominal pain and diarrhea [54] may occur in the early postoperative period. Long-term complications include tube obstruction and wound infection.

In some patients who are fed via a PEG tube, pulmonary aspiration may occur, and routine intrajejunal feeding has been suggested for these cases. An additional advantage is that bolus gastric tube feeding is more physiological, particularly with respect to insulin secretion. Furthermore, because the feeds can be given intermittently, it allows greater patient freedom (intrajejunal feeding should be given continuously rather than intermittently). Direct intrajejunal delivery of nutrients should probably be reserved for patients with gastroesophageal reflux, hiatus hernia, or recurrent aspiration on gastrostomy feeding.

Swallowing Therapy

Swallowing exercises are used to strengthen the orofacial musculature, maneuvers to improve poor laryngeal elevation and laryngeal closure during swallowing, and techniques to stimulate the swallow reflex. These methods are usually used before starting direct swallowing.

Exercises to enhance the function of the orofacial muscles are used to improve lip seal, mastication, and tongue movements. A simple technique known as "the supraglottic swallow" may improve the elevation and closure of the larynx during swallowing. During this maneuver, the subject holds his/her breath and swallows, and he/she releases the air by coughing. Patients with delayed or absent swallow reflex often benefit from thermal stimulation of the oropharyngeal receptors. The procedure has been claimed to improve triggering of the swallowing action and to reduce the bolus transit time. It involves the repeated application of a small laryngeal mirror dipped in ice to the anterior faucial arch. Sensitization may be repeated between swallows. Direct swallowing therapy can be started with small amounts of food (of the right consistency) under the supervision of a speech and language therapist when the risk of pulmonary aspiration is deemed to be low.

Surgical Treatment of Neurogenic Dysphagia

Cricopharyngeal myotomy is an effective method of treatment of dysphagia in patients with stroke, muscular dystrophy, and in patients with motor neuron disease. Careful selection of patients is essential prior to this procedure. Two important things should be looked for, that is, failure of relaxation of the pharyngeal sphincter must be demonstrated on videofluoroscopy. Secondly, the oral phase of swallowing, lip seal, voluntary initiation of swallowing, and the propulsive action of the tongue must also be preserved. Poor tongue movement (demonstrated on videofluoroscopy by the inability to propel or retrieve the food bolus) is a contraindication to cricopharyngeal myotomy. Patients with absent pharyngeal peristalsis or delayed triggering of the swallow reflex by 10 s or more are also unlikely to benefit from this treatment. Surgery for cricopharyngeal dysfunction after stroke and traumatic brain injury should be considered after the first 3 months of the disease onset.

Relaxation of the cricopharyngeus can also be achieved with "chemical cricopharyngeal myotomy" using botulinum toxin type A injections [55]. The location of the cricopharyngeal muscle is determined with direct esophagoscopy and electromyography (using a hooked wire electrode), and the toxin is injected transcutaneously into the dorsomedial part and into the ventrolateral part of the muscle on both sides. A total dose of botulinum toxin type A of 80–120 units is usually sufficient, and the mean beneficial effect of treatment is 5 months. This may be used in patients with lateral medullary syndrome.

References

1. Jones B, editor. Normal and abnormal swallowing: imaging in diagnosis and therapy. 2nd ed. New York: Springer; 2003.
2. Dodds WJ, Stewart ET, Logemann JA. Physiology and radiology of the normal oral and pharyngeal phases of swallowing. AJR Am J Roentgenol. 1990;154(5):953–63.
3. Logemann JA. Evaluation and treatment of swallowing disorders. 2nd ed. Austin: Pro-Ed; 1998.
4. Palmer JB, Rudin NJ, Lara G, Crompton AW. Coordination of mastication and swallowing. Dysphagia. 1992;7(4):187–200.
5. Hiiemae KM, Palmer JB. Food transport and bolus formation during complete feeding sequences on foods of different initial consistency. Dysphagia. 1999;14(1):31–42.
6. Dua KS, Ren J, Bardan E, Xie P, Shaker R. Coordination of deglutitive glottal function and pharyngeal bolus transit during normal eating. Gastroenterology. 1997;112(1):73–83.
7. Matsuo K, Hiiemae KM, Palmer JB. Cyclic motion of the soft palate in feeding. J Dent Res. 2005;84(1):39–42.
8. Buettner A, Beer A, Hannig C, Settles M. Observation of the swallowing process by application of videofluoroscopy and real-time magnetic resonance imaging-consequences for retronasal aroma stimulation. Chem Senses. 2001;26(9):1211–9.
9. Hodgson M, Linforth RS, Taylor AJ. Simultaneous real-time measurements of mastication, swallowing, nasal airflow, and aroma release. J Agric Food Chem. 2003;51(17):5052–7.
10. Palmer JB, Hiiemae KM. Eating and breathing: interactions between respiration and feeding on solid food. Dysphagia. 2003;18(3):169–78.
11. Palmer JB, Hiiemae KM, Liu J. Tongue-jaw linkages in human feeding: a preliminary videofluorographic study. Arch Oral Biol. 1997;42(6):429–41.
12. Mioche L, Hiiemae KM, Palmer JB. A postero-anterior videofluorographic study of the intraoral management of food in man. Arch Oral Biol. 2002;47(4):267–80.
13. Palmer JB. Bolus aggregation in the oropharynx does not depend on gravity. Arch Phys Med Rehabil. 1998;79(6):691–6.
14. Saitoh E, Shibata S, Matsuo K, Baba M, Fujii W, Palmer JB. Chewing and food consistency: effects on bolus transport and swallow initiation. Dysphagia. 2007;22(2):100–7.
15. Shaker R, Dodds WJ, Dantas RO, Hogan WJ, Arndorfer RC. Coordination of deglutitive glottic closure with oropharyngeal swallowing. Gastroenterology. 1990;98(6):1478–84.
16. Ohmae Y, Logemann JA, Kaiser P, Hanson DG, Kahrilas PJ. Timing of glottic closure during normal swallow. Head Neck. 1995;17(5):394–402.

17. Cook IJ, Dodds WJ, Dantas RO, et al. Opening mechanisms of the human upper esophageal sphincter. Am J Physiol. 1989;257(5 Pt 1):G748–59.
18. Ertekin C, Aydogdu I. Electromyography of human cricopharyngeal muscle of the upper esophageal sphincter. Muscle Nerve. 2002;26(6):729–39.
19. Shaw DW, Cook IJ, Gabb M, et al. Influence of normal aging on oral-pharyngeal and upper esophageal sphincter function during swallowing. Am J Physiol. 1995;268(3 Pt 1):G389–96.
20. Daniels SK, Foundas AL. Swallowing physiology of sequential straw drinking. Dysphagia. 2001;16(3):176–82.
21. Martin-Harris B, Brodsky MB, Michel Y, Lee FS, Walters B. Delayed initiation of the pharyngeal swallow: normal variability in adult swallows. J Speech Lang Hear Res. 2007;50(3):585–94.
22. Stephen JR, Taves DH, Smith RC, Martin RE. Bolus location at the initiation of the pharyngeal stage of swallowing in healthy older adults. Dysphagia. 2005;20(4):266–72.
23. Chi-Fishman G, Stone M, McCall GN. Lingual action in normal sequential swallowing. J Speech Lang Hear Res. 1998;41(4):771–85.
24. Chi-Fishman G, Sonies BC. Motor strategy in rapid sequential swallowing: new insights. J Speech Lang Hear Res. 2000;43(6):1481–92.
25. Chi-Fishman G, Sonies BC. Kinematic strategies for hyoid movement in rapid sequential swallowing. J Speech Lang Hear Res. 2002;45(3):457–68.
26. Daniels SK, Corey DM, Hadskey LD, et al. Mechanism of sequential swallowing during straw drinking in healthy young and older adults. J Speech Lang Hear Res. 2004;47(1):33–45.
27. Nishino T, Yonezawa T, Honda Y. Effects of swallowing on the pattern of continuous respiration in human adults. Am Rev Respir Dis. 1985;132(6):1219–22.
28. Nishino T, Hiraga K. Coordination of swallowing and respiration in unconscious subjects. J Appl Physiol. 1991;70(3):988–93.
29. McFarland DH, Lund JP. Modification of mastication and respiration during swallowing in the adult human. J Neurophysiol. 1995;74(4):1509–17.
30. Selley WG, Flack FC, Ellis RE, Brooks WA. Respiratory patterns associated with swallowing: Part 1. The normal adult pattern and changes with age. Age Ageing. 1989;18(3):168–72.
31. Klahn MS, Perlman AL. Temporal and durational patterns associating respiration and swallowing. Dysphagia. 1999;14(3):131–8.
32. Martin-Harris B, Brodsky MB, Michel Y, Ford CL, Walters B, Heffner J. Breathing and swallowing dynamics across the adult lifespan. Arch Otolaryngol Head Neck Surg. 2005;131(9):762–70.
33. Shaker R, Li Q, Ren J, et al. Coordination of deglutition and phases of respiration: effect of aging, tachypnea, bolus volume, and chronic obstructive pulmonary disease. Am J Physiol. 1992;263(5 Pt 1):G750–5.
34. Dozier TS, Brodsky MB, Michel Y, Walters Jr BC, Martin-Harris B. Coordination of swallowing and respiration in normal sequential cup swallows. Laryngoscope. 2006;116(8):1489–93.
35. Smith J, Wolkove N, Colacone A, Kreisman H. Coordination of eating, drinking and breathing in adults. Chest. 1989;96(3):578–82.
36. Matsuo K, Hiiemae KM, Gonzalez-Fernandez M, Palmer JB. Respiration during feeding on solid food: alterations in breathing during mastication, pharyngeal bolus aggregation and swallowing. J Appl Physiol. 1985;104(3):674–81. Epub 2007 Dec 27
37. Charbonneau I, Lund JP, McFarland DH. Persistence of respiratory-swallowing coordination after laryngectomy. J Speech Lang Hear Res. 2005;48(1):34–44.
38. Kidd D, Lawson J, Nesbitt R, et al. Aspiration in acute stroke: a clinical study with videofluoroscopy. Q J Med. 1993;86:825–9.
39. Celifarco A, Gerard G, Faegenburg D, et al. Dysphagia as the sole manifestation of bilateral strokes. Am J Gastroenterol. 1990;85:610–3.
40. Buchholz DW. Clinically probable brain stem stroke presenting as dysphagia and nonvisualised by MRI. Dysphagia. 1993;8:235–8.
41. Smithard DG, O'Neill PA, Martin DF, et al. The natural history of dysphagia following stroke. Dysphagia. 1997;12:188–93.

42. Coates C, Bakheit AMO. Dysphagia in Parkinson's disease. Eur Neurol. 1997;38:49–52.
43. Riski JE, Horner J, Nashold BS. Swallowing function in patients with spasmodic torticollis. Neurology. 1990;40:1443–5.
44. Wyllie E, Wyllie R, Cruse RP, et al. The mechanism of nitrazepam-induced drooling and aspiration. N Engl J Med. 1986;14:35–8.
45. Hockman CH, Bieger D. Inhibitory effect of diazepam on reflexly-induced deglutition. Proc Can Fed Biol Sci. 1979;2:85.
46. Nathadwarawala KM, Nicklin J, Wiles CM. A timed test of swallowing capacity for neurological patients. J Neurol Neurosurg Psychiatry. 1992;55:822–5.
47. Collins MJ, Bakheit AMO. Does pulse oximetry reliably detect aspiration in dysphagic stroke patients? Stroke. 1997;28:1773–5.
48. Ekberg O. Posture of the head and pharyngeal swallowing. Acta Radiol. 1986;27:691–6.
49. Drake W, O'Donoghue S, Bartram C, et al. Eating in side lying facilitates rehabilitation in neurogenic dysphagia. Brain Inj. 1997;11:137–42.
50. Goulding R, Bakheit AMO. Evaluation of the benefits of monitoring fluid thickness in the dietary management of dysphagic stroke patients. Clin Rehabil. 2000;14:119–24.
51. Park RHR, Allison MC, Lang J, et al. Randomised comparison of percutaneous endoscopic gastrostomy and nasogastric tube feeding in patients with persisting neurological dysphagia. BMJ. 1993;304:1406–9.
52. Wilson PS, Johnson AP, Bruce-Lockhart FJ. Videofluoroscopy in motor neurone disease prior to cricopharyngeal myotomy. Ann R Coll Surg Engl. 1990;72:375–7.
53. Ciocon JO, Silverstone FA, Graver LM, et al. Tube feeding in elderly patients. Indications, benefits and complications. Arch Intern Med. 1988;148:429–33.
54. Keohane PP, Attrill H, Love M, et al. Relation between osmolality of diet and gastrointestinal side effects in enteral nutrition. BMJ. 1984;288:678–80.
55. Schneider I, Thumfart WF, Potoschnig C, et al. Treatment of dysfunction of the cricopharyngeal muscle with botulinum A toxin: introduction of a new non-invasive method. Ann Otol Rhinol Laryngol. 1994;103:31–5.

Medical Management of Swallowing Disorders

8

Simran Singh

Introduction

Dysphagia or difficulty in swallowing is a problem in all age groups but more so in the elderly. It can be either primarily oropharyngeal or esophageal in origin. Patients with oropharyngeal dysphagia can present with symptoms of coughing or choking with swallowing, food sticking in throat, drooling, nasal regurgitation, weight loss, and episodes of recurrent pneumonia. Esophageal dysphagia can lead to sensation of food sticking in chest, oral or pharyngeal regurgitation, food sticking in throat, drooling, and weight loss [1]. Elderly population with dysphagia has a higher risk of malnutrition, nonhealing wounds, bed sores, and aspiration pneumonia [2]. This is especially common in patients with dysphagia due to neurological diseases, neurodegenerative diseases, or brain injury. A study using Subjective Global Assessment to assess nutritional status found that 16 % of patients with dysphagia related to brain disorders had concomitant malnutrition whereas 22 % of patients with neurodegenerative diseases had associated malnutrition [3].

Certain drugs can exacerbate dysphagia and patient's drug history should therefore be reviewed. Neuroleptics, benzodiazepines, anticonvulsants, antiparkinsonian drugs, diuretics, antihistaminics, antineoplastics, NSAID, and theophylline are some of the group of drugs which can worsen dysphagia.

This chapter will focus on the following causes of dysphagia:

1. *Motor causes*:
   Achalasia cardia
   Diffuse esophageal spasm
   Nutcracker esophagus

S. Singh
Internal Medicine and Intensive Care,
PD Hinduja National Hospital, Mahim, Mumbai 400016, India
e-mail: simransingh@hotmail.com

© Springer India 2015
G. Mankekar (ed.), *Swallowing – Physiology, Disorders, Diagnosis and Therapy*,
DOI 10.1007/978-81-322-2419-8_8

141

2. *Infectious esophagitis* more commonly with *Candida*, CMV, and HSV 1 is seen in patients with diabetes, HIV, hematological malignancies, and immunosuppressive therapies
3. *Drug-induced esophagitis*
4. *Connective tissue disorders:*
   Scleroderma, rheumatoid arthritis, Sjögren's
5. *Eosinophilic esophagitis*
6. *Post-intensive care dysphagia*

Gastroesophageal Reflux Disease

GERD (Fig. 8.1) is passive reflux of gastric contents into esophagus which causes symptoms or histopathologic changes in the esophagus or both.

Reflux occurs due to increased relaxation of lower esophageal sphincter allowing a spontaneous reflux or increased abdominal pressure (stress reflux). Whereas some reflux is normal, several factors may predispose patients to pathological reflux, including hiatus hernia [4], lower esophageal sphincter hypotension, loss of esophageal peristaltic function [5], increased compliance of gastric hypersecretory states, delayed gastric emptying, and overeating [6]. GERD can often be due to the presence of multiple factors.

A consistent paradox in gastroesophageal reflux disease is the imperfect correspondence between symptoms attributed to the condition and endoscopic features

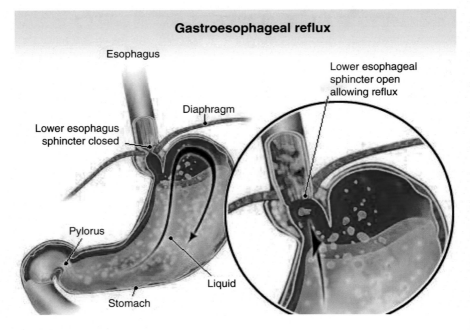

Fig. 8.1 Gastroesophageal reflux

of the disease. In a population-based endoscopy study in which 1,000 Northern Europeans were randomly sampled, the prevalence of Barrett's esophagus was 1.6 % and that of esophagitis was 15.5 % [7]. Although gastroesophageal reflux is the most common cause of heartburn, other disorders, e.g., achalasia and eosinophilic gastritis, may also contribute to the condition [8].

GERD with esophageal changes seen on endoscopy is known as endoscopy-positive GERD, while a disease with no demonstrable esophageal changes is known as endoscopy-negative or nonerosive reflux disease.

Contributory or Predisposing Factors for GERD

1. Obesity: there is a direct correlation between high body mass index and frequency and severity of GERD.
2. Pregnancy: during pregnancy the lower esophageal sphincter pressure reduces, and with increasing abdominal pressure, the risk of GERD increases.
3. Hiatal hernia: is an important risk factor for severe acid reflux.
4. Connective tissue disorders like scleroderma, mixed connective tissue disease, and Sjögren's and sicca syndrome can also give rise to GERD.

Clinical Presentation of GERD

Heartburn
Acid regurgitation
Indigestion/dyspepsia
Dysphagia
Epigrams trick pain
Abdominal bloating
Belching
Halitosis
Gastrointestinal bleeding
Wheezing/asthma
Nocturnal cough
Choking or aspiration of gastroesophageal contents
Atypical chest pain

Diagnostic Tests

When symptoms of gastroesophageal reflux disease are typical and the patient responds to therapy, no diagnostic tests are necessary to verify the diagnosis [9]. Diagnostic tests help to avert misdiagnosis; to identify any complications like a stricture, Barrett's metaplasia, or adenocarcinoma; and to evaluate treatment failures.

Important alternative diagnoses to consider include coronary artery disease, gall-bladder disease, gastric or esophageal cancer, peptic ulcer disease, esophageal motility disorders, and eosinophilic esophagitis.

1. Complete blood count to look for iron deficiency.
2. ECG for patients older than 45–50 years.
3. Upper gastrointestinal endoscopy is a standard test to look for esophagitis and peptic ulcer disease. If Barrett's esophagus or esophagitis (eosinophilic or *H. pylori* gastritis) is suspected, then endoscopic biopsies can be taken.
4. Esophageal manometry and 24 h ambulatory pH monitoring are indicated for persistent and refractory symptoms.
5. Gastric emptying scintigraphy – a nuclear medicine test can help in identifying patients who have gastroparesis causing a refractory GERD or those who are candidates for fundoplication.
6. Acid suppression test can be done by giving a trial of proton pump inhibitors.
7. Combined impedance-pH monitoring where quantifying exposure to esophageal acid and identifying reflux events regardless of acidic content are determined to establish GERD [10].

Treatment of GERD

1. Lifestyle modification: losing weight, avoiding foods that aggravate GERD, large meals, and alcohol should also be avoided.
2. H_2-receptor antagonists for symptomatic relief.
3. Proton pump inhibitors – help by reducing gastric acid secretion and are more effective than H_2 blockers. They provide symptomatic relief and prevent recurrence. In a large meta-analysis of 136 randomized controlled trials involving more than 35,000 patients with esophagitis, the rate of healing among patients treated with proton pump inhibitors (83 %) was greater than that with H_2 antagonists (52 %), and both rates were higher than a placebo [11]. In all trials, there were no major differences in efficacy noted among various proton pump inhibitors when used in standard doses.
4. Some patients with nighttime reflux benefit with a H_2 antagonist at night and a PPI in the morning.
5. Surgery to correct reflux is reserved for patients with severe symptoms that are refractory to treatment or if it is a complicated GERD, e.g. Barrett's esophagus, esophageal bleeding, or aspiration.
   Fundoplication, in which the proximal stomach is wrapped around the distal esophagus to create an antireflux barrier, is an alternative approach to chronic gastroesophageal reflux disease. Follow-up of patients who have received medical therapy as compared with surgery have shown no significant differences in the prevalence of Barrett's esophagus or in the prevalence of an adenocarcinoma [12].

Infectious Causes of Dysphagia

Infectious esophagitis is most commonly seen in immunocompromised patients. Fungal and viral diseases are the most common agents in this population. There are some rare instances where infectious esophagitis is seen in immunocompetent patients. Approximately 30 % of HIV patients have viral or fungal esophagitis during the course of their illness. Patients on chemotherapy, posttransplant patients on immunosuppressants, malignancies, head and neck radiation, and antibiotic exposure inhaled steroids are the other risk factors for infectious esophagitis.

Etiology

1. *Fungal Esophagitis:*
   Candidiasis (Fig. 8.2) is the most common infectious disease of the esophagus in patients with HIV accounting for 70 % of the cases. *Candida albicans* is most common species but other species have also been implicated.
2. *Viral Esophagitis:*
   - *Cytomegalovirus* is the most common cause of viral esophagitis (Fig. 8.3) in HIV patients and is seen if the CD_4 count is less than 100.
   - *Varicella zoster* can cause severe esophagitis in immunocompromised hosts. It can be seen in children with chickenpox or adults with herpes zoster infection.

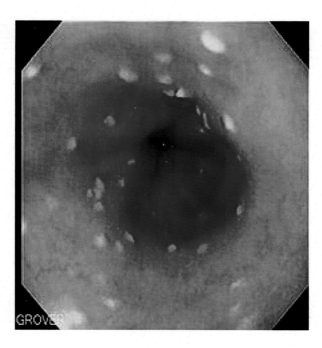

Fig. 8.2 Endoscopic image of esophageal candidiasis in a patient on chemotherapy

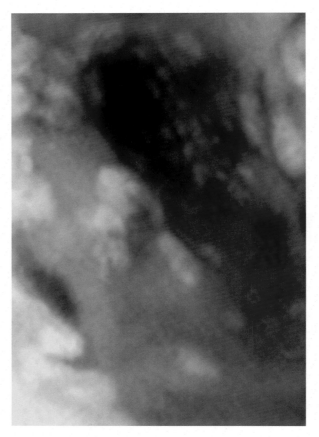

Fig. 8.3 Endoscopy picture of CMV-associated esophagitis before ganciclovir treatment (*Journal of Clinical Microbio* 2009)

- *Herpes simplex virus* is an uncommon cause of esophagitis (Fig. 8.4) in both immunocompetent and immunocompromised patients. It can be either a primary infection or more commonly reactivation of a latent virus in the distribution of the superior cervical, vagus, or laryngeal nerves [13].
3. *Bacterial* causes for esophagitis is rare even in HIV patients.
   Causative organisms could be *Mycobacterium avium-intracellulare*, *Mycobacterium tuberculosis*, and *Nocardia*

Clinical Presentation

Clinical presentation will depend upon the etiology of infectious esophagitis. In case of candidiasis, dysphagia is the most common symptom. Patients may also have oral thrush. Odynophagia, fever, and vomiting are less common. In case of

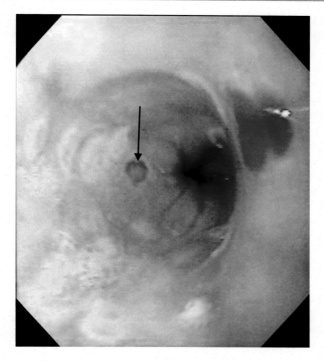

Fig. 8.4 Focal ulcerations (*arrow*) are typical of herpes simplex virus esophagitis (Picture courtesy MERCK Manual)

Cytomegalovirus, odynophagia and chest pain are more commonly associated with low-grade fever and vomiting. *Herpes simplex virus* presents with both dysphagia and odynophagia as well as pain and fever. Esophagogastroduodenoscopy can differentiate between different types of infections either grossly or on histopathologic appearance of the lesions [14].

Treatment for Infective Esophagitis

Treatment focuses on eradicating the causal organism.

1. *Esophageal Candidiasis:* Fluconazole – 200 mg loading dose followed by 100 mg OD for 5–10 days. In azole-resistant *Candida*, oral dose of fluconazole can be increased or echinocandins can be initiated.
2. *Cytomegalovirus Esophagitis:* Intravenous ganciclovir is the drug of choice. Alternate therapy is intravenous foscarnet. Treatment can continue for at least a month. Relapses are common.
3. *HSV Esophagitis:* Acyclovir 5 mg/kg IV, three times a day for 7–14 days, is the drug of choice.

Drug-Induced Esophageal Injury Leading to Swallowing Disorders

Medication-induced esophageal injury can occur at any age with a variety of commonly used medications. Most of the medications are over-the-counter medicines. These can be divided into those that cause direct injury to esophageal mucosa [15] and those that may contribute to the toxicity due to the contact time of the pill. Cellulose fiber and guar gum pills may swell and lodge in the esophagus causing complete obstruction.

Medication-induced esophagitis may be due to an underlying anatomic or motility disorder of the esophagus, allowing for a prolonged exposure of the drug to esophageal mucosa. Patients with esophageal stricture, left atrial enlargement, esophageal dysmotility, and esophageal diverticuli have a greater risk of drug-induced esophagitis.

Specific Medications Associated with Esophagitis (Table 8.1)

1. *Antibiotics:* Clindamycin, doxycycline, penicillin, rifampin, and tetracycline are some of the antibiotics associated with esophagitis.
2. *Nonsteroidal Anti-inflammatory Drugs:* Aspirin, ibuprofen, and naproxen [16].
3. *Other medications* like ascorbic acid, ferrous sulfate, lansoprazole, potassium chloride, and quinidine.
4. *Antiviral* agents particularly those used for treatment of HIV have also been reported to cause medication-induced esophageal injury. These include zalcitabine, zidovudine, and nelfinavir [17, 18].
5. *Biphosphonates:* This class of drugs is one of the commonest causes of medication-induced esophagitis. The injury has mainly been reported with alendronate, pamidronate, and etidronate. Risedronate has low potential for causing esophageal injury because of the rapid esophageal transit and therefore minimal contact with esophageal mucosa [19–21].

   Overall the incidence of injury is small but it can be serious and even fatal. Unfortunately reflux-type symptoms are common and can be difficult to differentiate from medication-induced mucosal injury [22].

   Diagnosis can be made endoscopically with marked exudates, inflammation, stricture formation, hemorrhage, and esophageal perforation being seen.

Table 8.1 Some of the esophagitis-inducing orally administered medications

Doxycycline
Tetracycline
Alendronate
Aspirin
Naproxen
Potassium chloride
Ascorbic acid
Iron sulfate
Quinidine

6. *Chemotherapy-Induced Esophagitis*

Dactinomycin, bleomycin, cytarabine, daunorubicin, 5-flurorouracil, methotrexate, and vincristine are some of the agents that can cause severe odynophagia, as a result of oropharyngeal mucositis. These drugs can also involve the esophagus but esophageal damage is uncommon in the absence of oral changes [23]. Treatment is aimed at symptom control, prevention of superimposed injury from acid reflux, maintenance of adequate hydration, and removal of offending medication. For symptom control, topical local anesthetics like viscous lidocaine solution can be given. Prevention of superimposed reflux is best treated by giving twice daily proton pump inhibitor. For patients with severe odynophagia, prohibiting oral intake and giving intravenous hydration may be necessary for a few days.

Also proper administration of potentially injurious medications will help avoid occurrence of esophageal injury. On the basis of sometimes normally slow transit of medications through the esophagus particularly for gelatin capsules and larger tablets, it is recommended that medications should be ingested with 8 oz of water, patients should remain upright for half an hour, and patients with underlying potential risk for esophageal injury should look for alternative, safer medicines [24].

Achalasia (Fig. 8.5)

Achalasia is characterized by impaired lower esophageal sphincter relaxation with swallowing and aperistalsis in the smooth muscle esophagus. The resting lower esophageal pressure is elevated in about 60 % of the cases [25].

These physiologic alterations result from damage to innervation of smooth muscle segment of the esophagus.

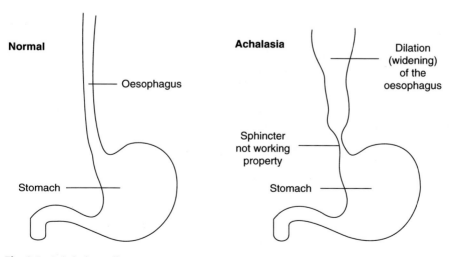

Fig. 8.5 Achalasia cardia

The neuroanatomic changes responsible for achalasia include loss of ganglion cells within the myenteric plexus and degeneration of vagus nerve and its dorsal motor nucleus. Of all these three possibilities, loss of ganglion cells is well substantiated [26]. The cause of ganglion cell degeneration in achalasia is pointing towards an autoimmune process caused by a latent HSV-1 infection in genetically susceptible individuals [27, 28].

Immunohistochemical analyses of the myenteric plexus infiltrate in these patients reveal that the majority of inflammatory cells are either resting or activated cytotoxic T cells [29]. Achalasia may also be associated with degenerative neurological disorders such as Parkinson's disease. These patients were noted to have Lewy bodies in the degenerating ganglion cells of the myenteric plexus [30].

Clinical Features

Dysphagia is the main symptom of esophageal motility disorders.

The associated symptoms of heartburn, chest pain, odynophagia, regurgitation, hiccups, halitosis, and weight loss are suggestive of esophageal dysphagia. Patients generally experience dysphagia to solid foods and some do experience variable dysphagia to liquids.

With long-standing disease, there is progressive esophageal dilatation, and regurgitation becomes more frequent. Some of these patients also have bronchopulmonary complications [31].

Investigations

1. *Upper endoscopy* should be the first investigation for evaluating new-onset dysphagia as one can detect most structural causes of dysphagia and also obtain biopsies. It has its limitations in assessing extraluminal structures, abnormal esophageal motility, and subtle obstructing lesions.
2. *Contrast imaging* of the esophagus and oropharynx is useful for a functional evaluation of the oropharyngeal phase of swallowing.
3. *Barium esophagogram* can provide information on upper esophageal sphincter function, peristalsis, and bolus clearance through esophagogastric junction.
4. *Esophageal manometry* uses intraluminal pressure sensors within the esophagus to quantify the contractile characteristics of the esophagus and segregate it into functional regions. The manometric evaluation of deglutitive esophagogastric junction is probably the most important measurement made during clinical esophageal manometry.
5. *Intraluminal impedance* measurement is used to assess intraluminal bolus transit without using fluoroscopy. It can be combined with manometry to assess the efficacy of esophageal function in assessment of dysphagia.
6. *Sensory testing* of esophageal nerves can also be used to assess neuromuscular causes of achalasia [32].

Treatment for Achalasia (Table 8.2)

The definitive treatment for achalasia is disruption of the lower esophageal sphincter either surgically or with a pneumatic dilator. The main therapeutic options are between pneumatic dilatation and laparoscopic Heller myotomy. One controlled trial compared pneumatic dilatation to myotomy via thoracotomy. This study reported 95 % symptom resolution with myotomy and 52 % symptom resolution in the dilatation group, but this study was critiqued for the methodology in the pneumatic dilatation group [33]. The most frequent complication associated with pneumatic dilatation is perforation.

Pharmacological therapy acts as a temporary measure. These include:

1. *Smooth muscle relaxants* such as nitrates or calcium channel blockers, administered sublingually immediately prior to eating which can relieve dysphagia by reducing the LES pressure. The largest experience has been with isosorbide dinitrate and nifedipine. Isosorbide nitrate 5–10 mg sublingually prior to meals reduces LES pressure by 66 % for 90 min. Placebo-controlled trials have not been reported. Common side effect is mainly headache [34, 35].
2. *Calcium channel blockers* (diltiazem, verapamil, nifedipine) reduce LES pressure by 30–40 % for more than an hour [35, 36]. The largest clinical experience has been with nifedipine 10 mg sublingually given prior to meals. Nifedipine was better than placebo in 70 % of the patients for at least 6–18 months. Side effects of nifedipine include flushing, headaches, and orthostasis [34].
3. *Sildenafil* is a phosphodiesterase inhibitor. A double-blinded study found that 59 mg of sildenafil significantly reduced LES pressure as compared to placebo. The effect was seen at 15–20 min of consuming the drug and the effect lasted for less than an hour [37].

Table 8.2 Treatment for Achalasia

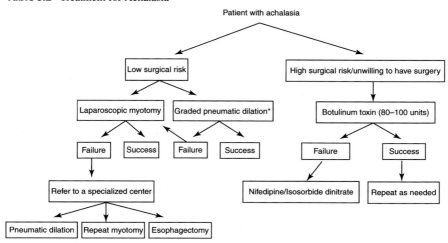

4. *Botulinum Toxin Injection:* Botulinum toxin irreversibly inhibits the release of acetylcholine from the presynaptic cholinergic receptors thereby eliminating the neurogenic component of LES pressure.

The initial study of botulinum toxin in achalasia reported that intrasphincteric injection of botulinum toxin decreased LES pressure by 33 % and improved dysphagia in 66 % of patients for a 6-month period [38]. Side effects included chest discomfort and rash. This treatment option is reserved for older adults who are poor risks for definitive treatments.

Eosinophilic Esophagitis (Fig. 8.6)

Eosinophilic esophagitis is being increasingly recognized as a cause of dysphagia, heartburn, and atypical chest pain that is unresponsive to antireflux measures. Its cause is unknown but allergic immune-mediated mechanisms similar to asthma and atopic diseases are implicated.

The disease is chronic and there is a high likelihood of symptom recurrence.

Eosinophilic esophagitis may be as common as inflammatory bowel disease.

The diagnosis is made by upper gastrointestinal endoscopy and esophageal biopsies showing eosinophilic infiltration. The growing incidence of eosinophilic esophagitis parallels that of other atopic diseases, e.g., asthma, eczema, and allergic rhinitis, raising the possibility that these disorders share a common environmental exposure and inflammatory pathways [39]. Complete evaluation for dietary

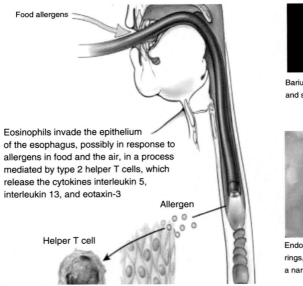

Food allergens

Eosinophils invade the epithelium of the esophagus, possibly in response to allergens in food and the air, in a process mediated by type 2 helper T cells, which release the cytokines interleukin 5, interleukin 13, and eotaxin-3

Allergen

Helper T cell

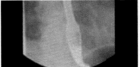

Barium studies may show focal narrowing and subtle concentric rings (trachealization)

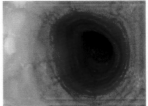

Endoscopy may reveal mucosal fragility rings, strictures, linear furrows, and a narrow caliber

Fig. 8.6 Eosinophilic esophagitis (Medical illustrator pangrace 2008)

allergens and aeroallergens is therefore recommended as avoidance of these can be helpful in some adults. Emerging data in adults suggests that a six-food elimination diet can improve symptoms and esophageal eosinophilia. The six foods most commonly associated with allergy are egg, wheat, soy, seafood, peanuts, and cow's milk protein. It is important to consult a nutritionist since elimination and elemental diet can result in important restrictions of calories and nutrients [40]. Acid reflux does not appear to be the primary causative factor in most patients. However, it may play a secondary role as some patients have experienced symptomatic, endoscopic, and histologic resolution of eosinophilic esophagitis after treatment with a proton pump inhibitor [41].

Spechler et al. [42] have suggested that mucosal injury caused by acid reflux may allow swallowed allergens to penetrate the esophageal layer that is otherwise impermeable to most proteins thereby causing eosinophilia. Conversely, the intense granulation of activated eosinophils seen in eosinophilic esophagitis can trigger changes in the lower esophageal sphincter which could lead to acid reflux.

The diagnosis of eosinophilic esophagitis is made histologically with marked eosinophilia on esophageal biopsies usually 15 or more per high-power field [43]. The recent consensus statement [43] recommends allergy testing. It states that between 50 and 80 % of patients with eosinophilic esophagitis have a coexisting atopic disease like asthma, eczema, dermatitis, or allergic rhinitis [43]. The prevalence is higher in children than in adults. In these patients, allergy testing will predict a response to treatment. Offending food or aeroallergens should be removed over a period of time, and during this time, patients should be monitored closely [43].

Medical Therapy

1. *Swallowed fluticasone* using an inhaler is the mainstay of treatment for both children and adults. Swallowed fluticasone is well tolerated although case reports of esophageal candidiasis have been reported.

   In one case series, 21 adult patients with eosinophilic esophagitis received a 6-week course of fluticasone 220 microgram/puff, two to four puffs/day. Symptoms completely resolved in all patients for at least 4 months and no patient needed esophageal dilatation [44].
2. *Acid Suppression:* It still has an unclear role in the treatment of eosinophilic esophagitis. The impact of concomitant therapy with proton pump inhibitor has not been determined, but the recent guidelines suggest that these drugs are reasonable as co-therapy in patients who also have GERD symptoms [43].
3. *Systemic corticosteroids* have been used for eosinophilic esophagitis, but adverse effects limit their long-term use.
4. *Mepolizumab:* Anti-IL-5 monoclonal antibody decreased the number of eosinophils in the esophagus and peripheral blood and improved clinical symptoms in an open-label trial [45].
5. *Endoscopic Dilatation:* Endoscopic dilatation with either a guide wire or a balloon technique is often used to treat strictures and a narrowed esophagus.

Diffuse Esophageal Spasm

DES occurs in 10–15 % of the patients with motility disorders.

Patients experience high-amplitude contractions in the smooth muscle portion of the esophagus. However, skeletal muscle function remains normal. The spastic waves are usually initiated by swallows but may occur randomly as well. The lower esophageal sphincter may have normal or high pressure and may not completely relax with swallowing [57]. Patients experience intermittent dysphagia to solids and liquids. DES is often confused with angina pectoris. Thus, it is important to exclude a possible cardiac disease. Treatment is directed towards decreasing the frequency and intensity of simultaneous contractions. Smooth muscle relaxants including nitrates, calcium channel blockers, psychotropic drugs, and anticholinergics have been tried with variable results. Pneumatic dilatation sometimes provides symptomatic relief. In difficult cases, surgical myotomy may be tried.

Nutcracker Esophagus (Fig. 8.7)

Nutcracker esophagus is a motility disorder in which the lower esophageal sphincter function and peristalsis are normal.

However, the contractile amplitude is two to three times the normal value. Most if these patients also have an abnormal prolongation of peristaltic wave. The symptoms and treatment of nutcracker esophagus are similar to diffuse esophageal spasm suggesting that these disorders are related.

Acquired Swallowing Disorders

Post-intensive Care/Extubation

Patients hospitalized in the intensive care unit (ICU) frequently develop swallowing disorders leading to aspiration, reintubation, pneumonia, and prolonged hospital stay. A significant portion of ICU patients who develop acute respiratory failure and require mechanical ventilation and survive to be extubated have dysfunctional swallowing, and it could be associated with poor patient outcomes [46]. These patients are also at a higher risk of developing critical illness poly-neuromyopathy, which may affect the bulbar as well as the peripheral muscles and nerves [47]. Neuromuscular weakness, local effects of endotracheal intubation, loss of normal sensation in the oropharynx and larynx, GERD, and altered sensorium could be some of the mechanisms contributing to ICU-acquired dysphagia. The diagnosis of swallowing disorders is made by a speech pathologist using a bedside swallowing evaluation [47].

The most common screening strategy is a water swallowing test with the nurse, physician, or the speech therapist observing the patient for signs of aspiration. It is the *3-oz bedside water swallow test*. Failure is not drinking the entire amount,

Fig. 8.7 Corkscrew
appearance of the esophagus
(Nutcracker esophagus
Hellerhoff – Own work.
Licensed under Creative
Commons. Wikipedia)

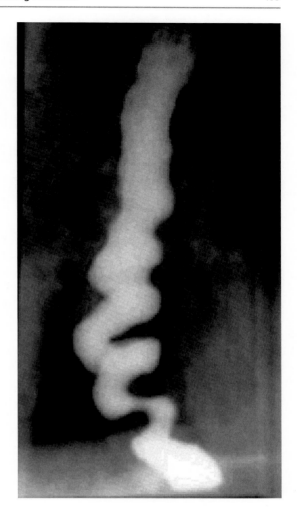

coughing, choking up to 1 min after the test, drooling, gurgling, and hoarseness. Anyone failing the three ounce water swallow test or those at higher risk for post-extubation failure should get a speech language pathology consultation [47]. More advanced tests to diagnose dysphagia after extubation can be carried out. They are:

1. Modified barium swallow (videofluoroscopic swallow study)
2. Endoscopy (fiberoptic endoscopic swallow study or FESS)

Treatments strategies (Table 8.3) include enteral feeding, controlling the texture of ingested food and liquids, speech and swallow therapy, respiratory therapy, monitoring dysphagia-causing drugs being administered, and periodic evaluation with FEES. In refractory cases, botulinum toxin injection, upper esophageal sphincter myotomy, or even feeding gastrostomy may be required [47].

Table 8.3 Algorithm for management post-intensive care/post-extubation dysphagia

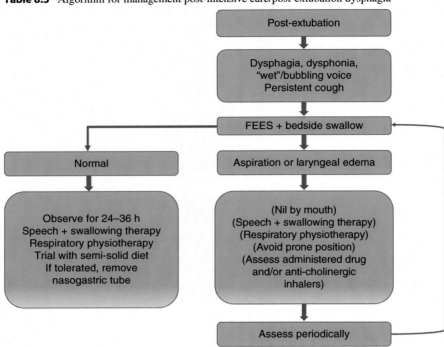

Swallowing Disorders Due to Musculoskeletal Diseases

1. *Scleroderma*

   Among the musculoskeletal diseases, dysphagia is best known as a complication of scleroderma, in which it is a feature of CREST syndrome. Although scleroderma can affect any part of the gastrointestinal system, the esophagus is involved most often with esophageal symptoms occurring in up to 90 % of the patients [48]. Dysphagia is rarely the presenting complaint of scleroderma.

   Usually the disease process involving the esophagus is quite diffuse. The smooth muscle layers of the esophagus are replaced by fibrous tissue leading to decreased peristalsis. The motility disturbance characteristically involves the body of the esophagus and the lower esophageal sphincter [49]. Incompetence of the lower esophageal sphincter can also contribute to the development of GERD. Reflux may be exacerbated by hiatus hernia which occurs in over 50 % of the patients due to dilatation and shortening of the esophagus [50].

   Impaired or absent esophageal peristalsis prevents clearance of reflux and prevents the acid from going back into the stomach [48]. Chronic acid reflux can lead to esophageal strictures, Barrett's metaplasia, and carcinoma. Esophagitis occurs in one-third of the patients, and its incidence increases to 100 % in patients with severe cutaneous involvement [51]. Poor emptying of the esophagus, immunosuppressive therapy, and acid suppression also predispose the patient to *Candida* esophagitis [52].

Other factors that may contribute to dysphagia in scleroderma include impaired mandibular motion and mastication due to atrophy and fibrosis of the perioral skin and reduced acid neutralizing capacity due to secondary Sjögren's syndrome [53].

2. *Sjögren's syndrome*

Dysphagia occurs in three-quarters of patients with Sjögren's syndrome and is related to lack of saliva and esophageal dysmotility [53].

Decreased or absent contractility has been shown in the upper third of the esophagus. The upper esophageal sphincter impairment may be more severe than in other connective tissue diseases [49].

3. *Systemic lupus erythematosus*

Dysphagia and heartburn are often seen in patients with SLE. Reduced esophageal motility is often seen in patients with SLE. Most commonly seen is abnormal peristalsis of the body of the esophagus [49].

Inflammation of the esophageal muscles or vascular damage to the Auerbach's plexus could be the possible reason for esophageal pathology.

4. *Rheumatoid arthritis*

Disorders of esophageal motility are found in 30 % of the patients with RA [54].

GERD and decreased peristalsis in the lower third of the esophagus is commonly seen although less frequently as compared to systemic sclerosis. Sicca syndrome and temporomandibular joint involvement may also make chewing and swallowing difficult [55].

Dysphagia has also been reported as a complication of laryngeal involvement with synovitis and nodules in RA and due to Plummer-Vinson syndrome in patients with RA and iron deficiency anemia [56].

Esophageal smooth muscle dysfunction is quite common in connective tissue diseases but is generally asymptomatic in the initial stages of the primary disease.

Summary

Oropharyngeal and esophageal dysphagia warrant urgent evaluation to determine the underlying etiology and to assess the severity of dysfunction prior to initiating treatment.

A videofluorographic swallowing study is useful for identifying the pathophysiology of a swallowing disorder and for empirically testing therapeutic and compensatory techniques. Manometry and endoscopy may also be necessary. Disorders of oral and pharyngeal swallowing are usually amenable to rehabilitative measures, which may include dietary modification and training in specific swallowing techniques. Surgery is rarely indicated. The goal of management of any form of dysphagia is to improve food transfer and prevent aspiration and of course to treat primary disease process as well.

References

1. Castell DO, Donner MW. Evaluation of dysphagia: a careful history is crucial. Dysphagia. 1987;2:65–71.
2. Palmer JB, et al. Evaluation and treatment of swallowing impairments. Am Fam Physician. 2000;61(8):2453–62.
3. Crary MA, Groher ME. Introduction to adult swallowing disorders. Philadelphia: Butterworth Heinemann; 2003.
4. DeVries DR, et al. Gastroesophageal reflux disease, relation with hiatal hernia, body mass index, esophageal acid exposure. Am J Gastroenterol. 2008;103:1349–54.
5. Corley DA, Kubo A, Levin TR, et al. Abdominal obesity and body mass index at risk patients for Barett's esophagus. Gastroenterology. 2007;133:34–41.
6. Hirshowitz BI, Simmons J, et al. Risk factors for esophagitis in extreme acid hyper secretion with or without Zollinger-Ellison syndrome. Clin Gastroenterol Hepatol. 2004;2:220–9.
7. Dellon ES, Shaeen NJ. Does screening for Barrett's esophagus and adenocarcinoma prolong survival? J Clin Oncol. 2005;23:4478–82.
8. Vakil N, Van Zarter SV, Kahriks P, et al. The Montreal Definition and classification of GERD: a global evidence based consensus. Am J Gastroenterol. 2006;101:1900–2000.
9. Armstrong D, Marshall JK, Chiba N, et al. Canadian Consensus Conference on the management of gastroesophageal reflux disease in adults. Update 2004. Can J Gastroenterol. 2004;19:15–35.
10. Kahrilas PJ, Shaeen NJ, Vaezi M. Management of gastroesophageal reflux disease. Gastroenterology. 2008;135:1392–413.
11. Khan M, Santana J, Donellan C, Preston C, Moayyedi P. Medical treatments in the short term management of reflux esophagitis. Cochrane Database Syst Rev. 2007;2:CD003244.
12. Shaeen N, Ransohoff DF. Gastroesophageal reflux, Barrett's esophagus and esophageal cancer: scientific review. JAMA. 2002;287:1972–81.
13. Sethumadavan S, Ramanathan J, Rammouni R, et al. An overview. Am J Gastroenterol. 2001;96:226.
14. Baehr PH, McDonald GB. Esophageal infections: risk factors, presentations, diagnosis and treatment. Gastroenterology. 1994;106:509.
15. Mc Cord GS, Clouse RE. Pill-induced esophageal structures. Clinical features and risk factors for development. Am J Med. 1990;88:512.
16. Bova JG, Dutton NE, Godstein HM, et al. Medication -induced esophagitis: diagnosis by double-contrast esophagography. Am J Roentgenol. 1987;148:731.
17. Edwards P, Turner J, Gold J, et al. Esophageal ulceration induced by zidovudine. Ann Intern Med. 1990;91:27.
18. Indorff A, Pergram PS. Esophageal ulceration related to zalcitabine. Ann Intern Med. 1992;117:133.
19. De Groen PC, Lubbe CF, Hirsch LJ, et al. Esophagitis associated with the use of alendronate. N Engl J Med. 1996;335:1016.
20. Macebo G, Azevedo F, Riberio T. Ulcerative esophagitis caused by etidronate. Gastrointest Endosc. 2001;53:250.
21. Licking EG, Argueta R, Whitaker MD, et al. Pamidronate: an unrecognised problem in gastrointestinal tolerability. Osteoporos Int. 1994;4:320.
22. Kikendall JW. Pill- induced esophageal injury. In: Castell DO, Richter JE, editors. The esophagus. 4th ed. Philadelphia: Lippincott Williams & Wilkins; 2004. p. 572.
23. Schubert MM, Peterson DE, Lloid ME. Oral complications in hematopoietic cell transplantation. 2nd ed. Cambridge: Blakwell Science; 1999. p. 751.
24. Hey H, Jorgensen F, Sirensen K, et al. Esophageal transit of six commonly used tablets & capsules. BMJ. 1982;285:1717.
25. Pandolfino JE, Kwiatek MA, Nealis T, et al. Achalasia: a new clinically relevant classification by high resolution Manometry. Gastroenterology. 2008;135:1526–33.

26. Csendes A, Smok G, Braghetto I, et al. Gastroesophageal sphincter pressure and histologic changes in distal esophagus in patients with achalasia. Dig Dis Sci. 1985;30:941–5.
27. Boeckxstaens GE. Achalasia: virus- induced euthanasia of neurons. Am J Gastroenterol. 2008;103:1610–2.
28. Facco M, Brun P, Baesso I, et al. T Cells in my enteric plexus of achalasia patients show a skewed TCR repertoire and react to HSV-1 antigens. Am J Gastroenterol. 2008;103:1598–609.
29. Clark SB, Rice TW, Tubbs RR, et al. The nature of myenteric infiltrate in achalasia. An immunohistochemical analysis. Am J Surg Pathol. 2000;24:1153–8.
30. Qualman SJ, Haupt HM, Yang P, Hamilton SR. Esophageal Lewy bodies associated with ganglion cell loss in achalasia. Gastroenterology. 1986;90:924–9.
31. Vantrappen G, Hellemans J. Treatment of achalasia and related motor disorders. Gastroenterology. 1980;79:144–54.
32. Drewes AM, Gregersen H. Multimodal pain stimulation of gastrointestinal tract. World J Gastroenterol. 2006;12:2477–86.
33. Richter JE. Surgery or pneumatic dilatation for achalasia. A head to head comparison. Gastroenterology. 1989;97:1340–1.
34. Bortoletti M, Labo G. Clinical and manometric effects of patients in with esophageal achalasia. Gastroenterology. 1981;80:39–44.
35. Gelfond M, Rozen P, Gilat T. Isosorbide dinitrate and nifedipine treatment of achalasia. A clinical and manometric and radionuclide evaluation. Gastroenterology. 1982;83:963–9.
36. Traube M, Hongo M, Magyar L, McCallum RW. Effects of nifedipine in achalasia and in patients with high amplitude peristaltic esophageal contractions. JAMA. 1984;252:1733–6.
37. Bortolotti M, Mari C, Lopilato C, et al. Effects of sildenafil on esophageal motility of patients with idiopathic achalasia. Gastroenterology. 2000;118:253–7.
38. Pasricha PJ, Ravich WJ, Hendrix TR, et al. Intrasphincteric botulinum toxin for the treatment of achalasia. N Engl J Med. 1995;332:774–8.
39. Rothenberg ME. Eosinophilic gastrointestinal disorders. J Allergy Clin Immunol. 2004;113:11–28.
40. Lucendo AJ, Arias Á, González-Cervera J et al: Empiric 6-food elimination diet induced and maintained prolonged remission in patients with adult eosinophilic esophagitis: a prospective study on the food cause of the disease. J Allergy Clin Immunol. 2013;131(3):797–804. doi:10.1016/j.jaci.2012.12.664. Epub 2013 Jan 31.
41. Ngo P, Furuta G, Antonioli D, Fox V. Eosinophils in the esophagus- peptic or allergic eosinophilic esophagitis? Case series of three patients with esophageal eosinophilia. Am J Gastroenterol. 2006;101:1666–70.
42. Spechler SJ, Genta RM, Souza RF. Thoughts on complex relationship between GERD and eosinophilic esophagitis. Am J Gastroenterol. 2007;102:1301–6.
43. Furuta GT, Liacouras CA, Collin MH, et al. Eosinophilic Esophagitis in children and adults: a systematic review and consensus recommendation for diagnosis and treatment. Gastroenterology. 2007;133:1342–63.
44. Arora AS, Perrault J, Smyrk TC. Topical corticosteroid treatment of dysphagia due to eosinophilic esophagitis in adults. Mayo Clin Proc. 2003;63:3–12.
45. Stein MK, Collins MH, Villanuaeva JM, et al. Anti-IL-5 therapy for eosinophilic esophagitis. J Allergy Clin Immunol. 2006;118:1312–9.
46. Macht M, Wimbish T, Benson AB, Burnham EL, et al. Post extubation failure is persistent and associated with poor outcomes in survivors of critical illness. Crit Care. 2011;15:R231.
47. Macht M, Wimbish T, Moss M. ICU-acquired swallowing disorders. Crit Care Med. 2013;41(10):2396–405.
48. Rose S, Young MA, Reynolds JC. Gastrointestinal manifestations of scleroderma. Gastroenterol Clin North Am. 1998;27:563–94.
49. Lapadula G, Muolo P, Semeraro F, et al. Esophageal motility disorders in rheumatic diseases: a review of 150 patients. Clin Exp Rheumatol. 1994;12:515–21.

50. Gareth JM, Winkleman RK, Schlegel JF, Code CF. Esophageal deterioration in scleroderma. Mayo Clin Proc. 1971;46:92–6.
51. Bassotti G, Battaglia E, Debernandi V, et al. Esophageal dysfunction in scleroderma: relationship with disease subsets. Arthritis Rheum. 1997;49:2252–9.
52. Ebert EC. Esophageal disease in scleroderma. J Clin Gastroenterol. 2006;40:769–75.
53. Sjogren RW. Gastrointestinal motility disorders in scleroderma. Arthritis Rheum. 1994;37:1265–82.
54. Janssen M, Dijkmans BAC, Lamers CBHW. Upper gastrointestinal involvement in rheumatoid arthritis patients: intrinsic or extrinsic pathogenesis? Scand J Gastroenterol. 1990;25 Suppl 178:79–83.
55. Sheehan NJ. Dysphagia and other manifestations of esophageal involvement in the musculoskeletal diseases. Rheumatology. 2008;47:746–52.
56. Medrano M. Dysphagia in a patient with rheumatoid arthritis and iron deficiency anaemia. MedGenMed. 2002;4:10.
57. Pehlivanov N, Liu J, Mittal RK. Sustained esophageal contraction: a motor correlate of heartburn symptom. Am J Physiol Gastrointest Liver Physiol. 2001;281:G743–51.

Pediatric Dysphagia

9

Justine Joan Sheppard and Georgia A. Malandraki

Introduction

The scope of pediatric dysphagia spans ages from birth to young adulthood. The functional concerns include sucking and swallowing in infancy; transition to semisolid purees; the acquisition and performance of mature, independent, eating behaviors that include biting, chewing, and drinking from cup and straw; and the progressive increase in efficiency of swallowing to support the increased calorie and hydration needs that are associated with growth [1]. This need for ongoing improvements in eating efficiency continues until the individual can sustain adult demands for nutrition and hydration. In addition, developmental competencies include sequences for increasing maturity in medications and saliva swallowing [2]. While the physiology of the oropharyngeal and esophageal phases of swallowing in children may differ somewhat from the adult, the concerns for timely initiation of the pharyngeal swallowing response, pharyngeal clearance, airway protection, and esophageal motility are similar.

When the ability to swallow is underdeveloped or impaired, the risk for disability or even death is greatly increased. Complications of pediatric dysphagia range from poor nutrition and growth and development failure to respiratory compromise, low weight, and increased mortality risk [3, 4]. Summaries of investigations on the

J.J. Sheppard
Department of Biobehavioral Sciences, Program of Speech and Language Pathology,
Teachers College, Columbia University, New York, NY, USA

Dysphagia Research Clinic, Edward D. Mysak Clinic for Communication Disorders,
Teachers College, Columbia University, New York, NY, USA

G.A. Malandraki, Ph.D., CCC-SLP, BCS-S (✉)
Department of Speech, Language and Hearing Sciences, Purdue University,
715 Clinic Drive / Lyles-Porter Hall Rm. 3152, West Lafayette, IN, 47907

Department of Biobehavioral Sciences, Teachers College, Columbia University, New York
e-mail: malandraki@purdue.edu

© Springer India 2015
G. Mankekar (ed.), *Swallowing – Physiology, Disorders, Diagnosis and Therapy*,
DOI 10.1007/978-81-322-2419-8_9

161

prevalence of feeding and swallowing disorders in children indicate that 33–80 % of children with developmental delays, 43–99 % of children with cerebral palsy (CP), and 46–89 % of children with autism spectrum disorders experience swallowing and feeding challenges [5–12]. Taking into consideration these large numbers, as well as the potentially devastating complications of swallowing and feeding disorders in a child's quality of life, health, and development, the need to optimally diagnose and treat them is crucial. The present chapter provides an overview of the main pathologies associated with pediatric dysphagia, the typical developmental course of feeding and swallowing, and the most widely used and evidence-based diagnostic and treatment modalities for this population.

Etiology and Pathophysiology in Pediatric Dysphagia

Pediatric dysphagia can be the result of a wide variety of conditions that can exist alone or in combinations. Although terminology differs, the major types of pediatric dysphagia can be thought of as developmental, neurological, mechanical/structural, medical, and behavioral. Under each of these categories, one can find many disease processes or mechanical deviations that cause pediatric dysphagia (Table 9.1). However, feeding and swallowing difficulties can also result from the interaction of two or more of these etiological factors/categories, necessitating diagnostic and therapeutic involvement from a multidisciplinary team [13].

Knowing the etiology underlying these difficulties is crucial for the accurate diagnosis of the swallowing disorder and treatment selection. The reason is that not all treatment options are appropriate for all pediatric patients. Oropharyngeal strengthening exercises may be ideal for children with reduced strength due to neurological or anatomical malformations but are traditionally contraindicated for children with increased spasticity in the head and neck. The pediatric swallowing specialist within a multidisciplinary team must be aware of the etiology causing the

Table 9.1 Main etiologies: categories of pediatric dysphagia and examples of some specific etiologies

Developmental	Neurological	Structural	Medical	Behavioral
Bronchopulmonary dysplasia	Pediatric CVA	Cleft lip/palate	GER(D)	Conditioned dysphagia
Developmental delay	TBI	Genetic syndromes	Allergies	post a medical
Intellectual	Brain tumors	Pierre Robin	EE	condition
disability	Neurosurgery	Velocardiofacial	Iatrogenic	Picky eaters
Down syndrome		syndromes	interventions	ASD
Cerebral palsy		Williams	Intubation	
		syndrome	Tracheostomy	
		Noonan		
		syndrome		
		Crouzon's		
		syndrome		

CVA cerebrovascular accident, *TBI* traumatic brain injury, *GER(D)* gastroesophageal reflux (disease), *EE* eosinophilic esophagitis, *ASD* autism spectrum disorders feeding and swallowing difficulties in order to provide appropriate treatment recommendations or referrals.

One of the main causes of developmental dysphagia can be prematurity. According to a recent systematic review on the causes of dysphagia across age groups, prematurity was the most commonly reported cause of dysphagia in newborns [14]. Prematurity (i.e., birth <37 weeks gestational age) means that the infant has to be able to breathe and feed before the aerodigestive systems are completely developed. In addition to this, in most situations the preterm infant also faces other medical conditions that may have to be treated invasively, exposing them to unpleasant experiences that further impact on feeding and swallowing development [15]. Frequently these factors lead to immature oral sensorimotor skills and inefficient sucking that can take considerable time and effort to remediate [16, 17]. Additionally, the preterm infant may present with respiratory compromise (bronchopulmonary dysplasia) contributing to difficulty coordinating the typical suck-swallow-breath cycle, a necessary skill for safe ingestion and airway protection [18].

Developmental dysphagia is also frequent in children with developmental delays and disorders that interfere with the developmental progression of swallowing and feeding skills (such as intellectual impairment, Down syndrome, or cerebral palsy) especially in the early years of life [5, 6, 11, 12, 19]. Developmental dysphagia in these populations typically is associated with impairments or delays in the development of mature eating skills as well as the complex of oropharyngeal sensorimotor swallowing functions [20].

Neurological etiologies affect the transmission of commands to and from the central nervous system resulting in impaired function of an otherwise normal structural oropharyngeal mechanism. In pediatric patients, typical neurological conditions that may affect or disrupt feeding and swallowing development include pre-, peri- and postnatal stroke leading to different forms and severity of cerebral palsy [5], traumatic brain injury [21], tumors affecting the brainstem and posterior fossa area [22], infant seizure disorders, and post-neurosurgical procedures [23]. Neurogenic dysphagia can manifest as difficulty in any of the swallowing phases but also is frequently accompanied by cognitive, alertness, language, and awareness deficits that can complicate symptoms and outcomes [24, 25].

Alternately, mechanical or structural abnormalities disrupt the anatomic or mechanical/physiological integrity of the oropharyngeal system leading to mechanical/structural dysphagia. Structural dysphagia in children can be congenital or acquired. Several structural abnormalities or conditions have been associated with feeding and swallowing difficulties in children. Some of the most common include cleft of the lip and/or palate and a variety of congenital genetic syndromes (such as Pierre Robin sequence, velocardiofacial syndromes, Williams syndrome, Noonan syndrome, Opitz BBB/G syndrome, etc.) that are frequently accompanied by developmental anomalies in one or more of the critical oropharyngeal and aerodigestive tract structures (nasal cavity, lips, mandible, tongue, palate, larynx, trachea, or esophagus) [26–29] [see authors' note 1 in Case Study Box]. Inadequate development of these structures may lead to swallowing difficulties ranging from inadequate ability to form a labial or palatal seal and reduced ability to suck or form and transfer a bolus to decreased airway protection [30].

Case Study Box
History

AB was a 5-year, 6-month-old male with a diagnosis of Opitz BBB/G syndrome and Asperger's syndrome. Anatomical anomalies in association with the Opitz BBB/G syndrome included level III laryngo-esophageal cleft, laryngomalacia, subglottic stenosis, and unilateral cleft of the upper lip and alveolar ridge, all of which were surgically corrected in the first 5 years of life. AB was also status post tracheostomy with tracheostomy decannulation occurring 10 months prior to the initiation of the program. AB had been totally dependent on gastrostomy tube (GT) feeding for nutrition and hydration since 3 weeks old. He had transitioned from GT feeding to a liquid diet taken only by straw in the last 2 weeks before our team saw him at age 5 or 6.

Authors' note 1: This is a typical example of a pediatric patient who experienced severe dysphagia due to a genetic syndrome causing multiple anatomic malformations. In addition, he has the behavioral characteristics of autism spectrum disorder. Post medical and surgical interventions, the child experienced conditioned dysphagia and avoidance behaviors that are often associated with prolonged interruption of oral feeding. Further, he had not had the opportunity to develop eating skills.

Feeding/Swallowing Evaluation

At the time of the evaluation, he fed himself a liquid-only diet at a rate of 32 mL/min; he was not accepting or swallowing puree or other solid foods and he was not eating from spoon or fork or drinking from an open cup. Thus, his oral feeding development was significantly delayed for his age. In addition, there were concerns with persistent aerophagia (i.e., excessive air swallowing), which became more apparent post decannulation and required frequent air suctioning from the GT to alleviate stomach distention and feelings of pain and discomfort. Although he had recurrent bouts of pneumonia in the past, he had been free from a pneumonia diagnosis for the past 3 months. Body Mass Index indicated that his nutrition was within normal limits for his age. A videofluoroscopic swallowing study (VFSS) was performed, which revealed no aspiration or penetration and no apparent oropharyngeal swallowing difficulties on the small boluses of liquids that he was able to swallow during the examination. Medications at baseline included azithromycin, Movicol, and Dulcolax. AB also had multiple food and environmental allergies. He had no apparent gross or fine motor deficiencies or difficulties, and speech and language appeared to be developing normally.

He was referred to our team for assistance with developing eating skills and tolerances for solid foods.

Authors' note 2: A clinical and instrumental evaluation was completed with this patient, as he exhibited significant oral feeding development delays and physiological symptoms (aerophagia), which needed to be examined clinically and instrumentally. The videofluoroscopic study revealed normal oropharyngeal swallowing, and thus the feeding program focused on the behavioral aspects of his dysphagia.

Treatment Program

Treatment focused on the following parameters that were found to be disordered during the evaluation: (1) oral acceptance/tolerance of eating-related objects and a variety of foods/flavors via spoon, (2) control of voluntary saliva swallows to improve aerophagia levels, (3) increase bolus size, and (4) increasing independence during feeding. The following techniques were used to address these parameters: (a) blocked sequence practice (e.g., AB was asked to practice one task at a time for multiple repetitions, then rest and practice again), (b) reduced response effort (e.g., AB practiced inserting a simulated spoon in his mouth prior to initiating spoon-feeding), (c) extrinsic feedback (e.g., frequent and immediate verbal acknowledgment of adequate performance was provided to AB for most tasks), (d) reinforcement (e.g., a sticker was given to AB after each successfully completed activity), and (e) new strategy "racing car swallow" to improve aerophagia and control of voluntary swallows (this was a strategy developed based on patient's interests in racing cars). We also used straw drinking (technique f), because this was a well-developed skill for AB to continue improving orobuccal coordination. Lastly, we encouraged AB to use a chin tuck posture (technique g) as an added safety precaution and a means for better assurance that he was using a propulsion swallow.

Authors' note 3: The techniques described above include examples of motor learning techniques (techniques a–e), one strengthening technique (technique f), and one compensatory strategy (technique g).

Oropharyngeal dysphagia in children can also result from a variety of medical conditions and/or procedures. Two of the most common medical conditions known to result in feeding and swallowing challenges include gastroesophageal reflux (GER) and allergies [31]. GER can be present in up to 85 % of infants and has been found to be more severe in high-risk neonates [32]. In most infants GER is considered a normal physiologic process that occurs several times per day and does not cause overt symptoms of discomfort [33]. In rare cases (about 5 %), it can persist beyond the first year of life. When GER progresses to GER disease (GERD), symptoms may range from feeding and sleeping difficulties, esophagitis, and pulmonary problems to failure to thrive and risk for aspiration [34]. Additionally, there is a high prevalence of GERD in children with intellectual and developmental disability that may present with rumination, vomiting, and behavioral issues [35]. GER can frequently coexist with food allergies including the frequent cow's milk protein allergy (CMPA). Food allergies and GER can cause discomfort and even pain during eating, experiences that can make eating undesirable for an infant or young child. Such conditions may further lead to conditioned dysphagia and avoidance behaviors during feeding in order for the child to avoid the discomfort and the pain [31]. Another related condition that appears to be frequently associated with dysphagia and feeding difficulties in children is eosinophilic esophagitis (EE). EE is a condition in which there is a dense infiltrate of eosinophils (white blood cells) on the esophageal mucosa, without the presence of GER [36]. The exact cause of EE is not well known; however, allergic causes [37] and some genetic predisposition have been reported [38]. Typical symptoms of EE include vomiting, dysphagia, feeding disorders, heartburn, and food impaction [37]. Additionally, children who have suffered from variable medical conditions, such as cardiac, orofacial, laryngeal, and pulmonary surgeries, or have experienced invasive medical procedures, such as intubation and tracheostomy, may develop analogous avoidance behaviors or even lack of appetite and motivation to eat, especially if eating has been interrupted for a long period of time or takes extra time and effort [29, 39–41]. Thus, medical dysphagia can easily result or manifest as behavioral dysphagia, which was conditioned aversions based on unpleasant experiences [see authors' note 1 in Case Study Box]. Typically, in these cases, there is delayed development of skills as well.

Behavioral dysphagia can result from some of the conditions described above or can be the result of neurodevelopmental disorders such as autism spectrum disorders (ASD) [42, 43]. Children with ASDs do not usually present with the typical inadequacies in oropharyngeal competencies described above but more commonly present with increased food selectivity regarding the type, brand, texture, temperature, or color of food (often called "picky eaters") [43, 44], a restricted dietary inventory [42], and in some cases atypical eating habits, such as tendency to eat inedible objects referred to as foreign body ingestion and pica [45, 46]. Additionally, adipsia and inability or refusal to ingest enough fluids have also been reported in cases with ASD and could potentially lead to further nutritional and gastrointestinal deficiencies [47]. These behaviors are often the result of a combination of sensory awareness and processing challenges potentially including all sensory modalities (gustatory, tactile, visual, auditory, proprioceptive, etc.), gastroesophageal difficulties (with GER being the most commonly reported), the urge for stereotypic behaviors, and executive function limitations, such as difficulties in planning or self-monitoring during the eating process [48].

For the medical professional who treats any of the aforementioned dysphagias, it is crucial to understand the normal development of feeding and eating behaviors and processes before they can offer a comprehensive diagnostic and therapeutic plan. Next we offer a concise review of the normal development of feeding and swallowing from the prenatal period to early childhood.

Normal Feeding and Swallowing Development

Understanding normal development is crucial in providing correct diagnosis and treatment in pediatric dysphagia. The rapid growth of technology has allowed for exciting opportunities for new knowledge on the development of swallowing and feeding in the pre- and postnatal periods.

Prenatal Period

Prenatally, the aerodigestive tract organs important for swallowing are developed during the embryonic period (weeks 1–8 of gestation) [49]. On the 3rd week of gestation, the three embryonic germ layers form (ectoderm, endoderm, mesoderm), which will later give rise to all the tissues and organs associated with swallowing. The digestive system develops between the 4th and 8th week of gestation, with the oropharynx including the tongue developing at the 5th week, followed by the labial muscles and the upper lip fusion by the 7th week of gestation [50]. Palatal development begins at the same time and is complete by the 12th week [51]. A combined laryngotracheal-esophageal tube starts separating by the 4th week of gestation providing a complete separation between the airway and the esophagus except for the level of the larynx. Thus, the esophagus starts developing at the 4th week; by week ten, it is lined by ciliated epithelial cells, and at 4 months, these cells start being replaced by squamous epithelial cells [52]. Respiratory and neural development initiates early but continues post the embryonic period and until birth [30]. The presence of immature taste buds on the tongue has been observed as early as the 7th week of gestation [53].

During the fetal period (9–28 weeks of gestation), there is continued rapid growth of structures and the first functions related to sucking and swallowing. Early oral movements, such as tongue thrusting and lip and jaw motions, have been noted as early as 15 weeks of gestation and are believed to be precursors for sucking and swallowing functions [54, 55]. These movements are seen to progress from simple open-close or anterior movements to the more complex repetitive movements typically seen in postnatal sucking. Swallowing has been observed as early as the 12th week of gestation, as the fetus swallows amniotic fluid. According to Miller and colleagues [56], bolus swallows more typically occur from 15 to 38 weeks gestational age (GA), with the most active period of swallowing occurring between 17 and 30 weeks GA [56]. Swallowing of amniotic fluid by the fetus is important in the regulation of the composition of the fluid and for the development of the gastrointestinal tract [57]. During these immature swallows, several functions, such as labial and velopharyngeal closure or even laryngeal elevation and airway closure, are not consistently observed [56, 58]. Swallowing in the fetus is also primarily seen in the presence of precedent oral-facial stimulatory activity, such as facial, ear, and labial swiping using the arm or hand, which starts as early as the 10th week of gestation [59]. Additionally, the taste buds typically develop into more morphologically mature taste buds by the 12th week [60]. There is preliminary evidence that the human taste system is functional in utero [61], although more research is needed in this area. According to Arvedson [62], a healthy preterm infant can suck and swallow functionally enough to maintain their nutritional needs with oral feeding by 34 weeks of gestation.

Postnatal Period: Infancy to 6 Months

Before we elaborate on the typical feeding and swallowing development in this period, we need to define two terms. The term "swallowing" refers to the complex sensorimotor sequence of events that are initiated by recognizing the presence (touch), taste, temperature, and viscosity of food or fluid in the oral cavity, followed by the preparation, in the case of food, to a consistency that can be swallowed, and finalized by its safe transportation through the oral, pharyngeal, and esophageal anatomic structures to the stomach [63]. "Feeding" refers to anticipatory events, such as motivation and readiness for eating, food acceptance, and also the important interactions developed between the infant and the caregiver/feeder during the feeding process [64]. How do these functions develop in the first months of life?

Normal feeding and swallowing milestones in infancy are achieved in parallel with other important psychosocial, sensorimotor, and cognitive development milestones. The full-term infant feels hunger and via infant oral reflexes (rooting reflex) searches for a breast or bottle nipple to initiate sucking and swallowing [62]. Healthy term and preterm infants can coordinate the sucking, swallowing, and breathing triad within 1–2 weeks post birth. According to Kelly and colleagues [65], any changes or irregularities seen in this coordination in the 1st weeks of life depend on neural or anatomical development or overall feeding experience.

The tongue and jaw plays a very important role in the execution of nutritive sucking (NS) (sucking conducted for nutritional purposes). Specifically, for the initiation of nutritive sucking, the tongue is known to either secure the nipple at the hard-soft palate junction and then initiate a downward movement for milk suction and upward movement for expression [66] or to be "anchored" at the anterior sulcus and initiate suction and expression movements [59]. Sucking may also be nonnutritive (NNS) occurring in infancy as an action on a hand or an object, usually a blocked nipple. In the premature infant, it occurs prior to readiness for NS. NNS in the infant is important for self-regulation, respiratory balance, feeding stability, and gastrointestinal health [67, 68]. A common scale used to evaluate sucking maturity in preterm and term infants involves five differential levels (Table 9.2) and was developed by Lau et al. (2000).

During the first months of feeding development, the infant has a flexed body posture, and his/her oral motor skills (such as lip closure, anterior-posterior movement of the tongue, and jaw range of motion) gradually improve. Simultaneously, several neuromotor and psychosocial milestones are achieved, including visual

Table 9.2 Stages of sucking development in preterm infants [69]

Sucking development stages
1a: No suction
1b: Arrhythmic alteration between suction and expression
2a: No suction; rhythmic expression
2b: Arrhythmic alteration between suction and expression, but also presence of sucking bursts
3a: No suction; rhythmic expression
3b: Rhythmic suction and expression; increase in suction amplitude, amplitude range, and duration of sucking bursts
4: Rhythmic suction and expression; suction is now well defined, decrease in amplitude range
5: Rhythmic, well-defined suction and expression; increase in suction amplitude; full-term infant sucking pattern

fixation, eye tracking [70, 71], more balanced body, neck and trunk support [72], ability to express hunger cues (through crying, arousal, sucking, etc.) [73], and increasing interaction between the feeder and the child that further facilitates a successful feeding experience. By 4 months, the infant can dissociate the lip and the tongue, and oral exploration is increased, as evidenced by increased labial movements, by performance of raspberries (bubbles formed with saliva and intense labial exploration by the infant), and by increased sound production [74]. By the 5th month, some infants are ready to initiate cup drinking [62]. Also, they now visually recognize objects and familiar faces and can use extended reach and grasp [71], and they are ready to initiate a more upright posture during feeding.

Six Months to 3 Years of Life

At around 6 months of life, transitional feeding is initiated, which includes the transition from bottle/nipple to spoon-feeding. The exact point in time when spoon-feeding is initiated depends on multiple environmental, neurodevelopmental, and feeding development factors. Specifically, Arvedson suggests that spoon-feeding readiness in the typically developing child depends on factors such as ability to maintain upright sitting posture and midline position of the head independently, hand to mouth movements, dissociation of labial and lingual movements, and anatomic head and neck changes that allow for more flexible lingual and jaw movements [62]. At about this time, the suck-swallow used for nipple feeding transitions from a swallow that depends on the gravity for transferring the bolus into the pharynx to one that depends on tongue propulsion. In the next few months (6–9 months), the child's oral and pharyngeal motor skills continue to mature, and the skill of eating thicker and lumpier foods develops, followed by finger feeding of easily dissolvable and soft chewable foods at 9–12 months and overall increased independence. A delay in the introduction of lumpy foods has been associated with reduced variety of foods accepted at later months of life and with increased incidence of feeding difficulties [75] and thus should be avoided. Chewing is rather stereotypical initially characterized by immature vertical movements caused by reciprocally activated antagonistic muscle groups [76] and gradually matures and requires less time and fewer chewing cycles [77]. Cup drinking is initiated at around the same time and may be challenging at first, but in most healthy children, this skill matures by the 15th month of age [73]. In addition to physiological readiness, the timing for acquisition of these skills depends on the introduction of foods and supports needed for practice of the skills [78].

By 13–18 months of life, healthy children are able to accept most textures, can coordinate phonation, swallowing and breathing rather well, and can initiate safe straw drinking [73]. By the second year of life, the child can self-feed adequately, a rotary chewing pattern has developed [77], and food intake is now independent. By the third year of life, most feeding and swallowing skills have acquired near-adultlike form, for unrestricted variety of food and liquid. The child eats with good jaw rotations as needed and complete mastication of the bolus and exhibits steady cup holding and drinking, use of fork, and total self-feeding [62].

Significant Considerations

The knowledge of normal development of feeding and swallowing skills is important in order to accurately evaluate differences and deviations in pediatric patients. Several considerations should be noted, however. First, the aforementioned milestones represent the course of feeding development for typically developing children, but a range of variability in the exact timing of acquisition of specific skills is to be expected. Differences may be seen because of cultural, geographical, or idiosyncratic reasons, and clinicians/physicians need to be aware of those. Additionally, according to Delaney and Arvedson, for preterm infants, clinicians should use age adjustments for the first 2 years of life before making determinations for diagnostic and therapeutic goals [64]. Development of feeding skills in preterm infants should be evaluated in the context of their adjusted age and general psychomotor development.

Another important consideration involves the concept of critical and sensitive periods in feeding development [79, 80]. These periods in relation to feeding mainly refer to the periods during which a child needs to transition from a simpler food type/consistency to a more advanced food type/consistency (mostly from liquids to solids). Although the exact range of months for the acquisition of each developmental skill is not absolute and can vary in normal infants and children, research has shown that children who are delayed in the introduction of new food consistencies (e.g., lumpy foods) will consume a reduced variety of foods later in life [75, 81] and that food acceptance is higher in children between 1 and 2 years of age and decreases significantly in the years following the second year of life [82]. This evidence supports the concept of critical/sensitive periods for feeding development. In addition, all the oropharyngeal, general motor, and respiratory physiological processes that govern feeding development also undergo critical/sensitive periods and should be considered [62]. In normally developing children, the parents should be encouraged to follow the typical feeding milestones described herein. In children with neurodevelopmental delays or disorders, however, additional factors including psychosocial, neuromotor, cognitive, medical, and general development should also be considered, before the determination to advance to a different food/consistency type is made.

Assessment Approaches

Clinical Dysphagia Assessment

As in the adult, dysphagia diagnosis in pediatrics may require a combination of clinical and instrumental assessments to fully evaluate the swallow and determine the contributing causes. Comprehensive classification systems have provided discrete categories of structural abnormalities, neurologic conditions, behavioral issues, cardiorespiratory problems, and metabolic disorders [7]. However, the clinical dynamic in pediatric dysphagia is most often a combination of physiologic, behavioral, and developmental features that are challenging for both diagnosis and treatment [13, 83, 84].

Screening Models

Subjective models that screen for referral for the CDE may include items that describe signs and symptoms of disorder or failed readiness for transitions. They may include, for example, prolonged (slow) feeding, respiratory signs associated with eating or saliva swallowing, repeated lower respiratory infections, persistent food refusal or restricted food preferences, irritability during meals, restricted food intake at meals, emesis associated with meals, interrupted or slow weight gain, failure to transition as expected to more mature eating patterns or foods and eating independence, and episodes of dehydration or choking [1, 2, 5, 83, 85].

Standardized screening assessments, tests that estimate presence, and may describe the clinical presentation, of disorder but do not address contributing causes, have been tested for pediatric applications. The 3-ounce water challenge was studied for its use to screen for aspiration. Children 2–18 years old able to drink 3 ounces of water by cup or straw were tested. Indications for failure were inability to drink the 3 ounces and coughing. Results indicated that there were adequate sensitivity and specificity for its use as a screening; however, further clinical assessment was needed for determining indicators for appropriate feeding status and diet [86]. The dysphagia disorder scale, a screening assessment for presence of dysphagia in children and adults with developmental disability, is administered during an observation of a meal or snack. Study results have found it to be a reliable and valid test for identifying and describing the clinical presentation of swallowing and feeding disorders. When used in conjunction with an ordinal scale, the dysphagia management staging scale, it provides a measure of functional severity of disorder [2, 87]. Parent-report inventories have been standardized for use in pediatric dysphagia for children with autism [88], for children who are tube fed [89], and for a range of problematic eating behaviors that include dysphagia [90, 91].

The Clinical Dysphagia Evaluation

The clinical dysphagia evaluation (CDE) is considered to be pivotal as a minimally invasive method for determining signs and symptoms of dysphagia. It is during the CDE that the clinician makes the preliminary determination of the dysphagia diagnosis and the categories of contributing cause and decides whether or not the condition warrants instrumental or collaborative team assessments to further delineate the parameters of the swallowing and feeding disorder. The CDE determines the clinically apparent signs and symptoms [84, 92, 93].

Subjective models for pediatric CDE may include the case history, examination of oral, pharyngeal, facial and thoracic anatomy, examination of oral and pharyngeal reflexes, and the observation of swallowing function for saliva, foods, and liquids. The case history can be extensive, including family, medical, nutritional, developmental, and feeding information that suggest possible etiologies, causes, and consequences of the complaint. During observations of infant reflex responses and swallowing and feeding function, the integrity of cranial nerve participation is analyzed. Judgments are made as to the adequacy of body postural control and alignment and breath support and swallow-breathing coordination. In pediatrics, considerations are included for developmental levels for eating milestones and for levels of independence, motivation for eating, and eating pragmatics. These diagnostic CDE models have been developed for infants and for older children [1, 2, 93, 94].

Objective clinical assessments have been developed for standardized observation of sucking in infants and oropharyngeal dysphagia in children. These assessments can be valuable as they have been shown to reduce clinician bias and provide levels of assurance of validity, reliability, and responsiveness. However useful these assessments may be, psychometric limitations have been noted [87, 95–98]. Generally, these assessments have been standardized for specific populations and specific feeding skills. Howe and colleagues reviewed dysphagia assessments that have been developed for preterm and term infants, for breastfeeding and bottle-feeding, and for evaluating infant function and maternal participation [95]. Benfer and colleagues reviewed assessments of oropharyngeal dysphagia that have been developed for children with cerebral palsy and neurodevelopmental disabilities. These assessments examine swallowing and feeding function variably in natural eating situations and with test items that include a range of solid and fluid foods [96, 99].

Ordinal scales have been developed for classifying levels of severity of swallowing and feeding disorder in cerebral palsy. Few are standardized [100, 101]. The ordinal parameters vary from overall measures of function to measures of specific competencies, e.g., food textures, assistance needed for eating, respiratory illness, and risk for aspiration. Standardized assessments for objectifying observations of specific, clinically apparent skills and for examining the behavioral milieu during eating have been useful in clinical practice and research. Examples of this type of clinical assessment are an observation of mother-infant interaction and an observation of mastication [89, 91, 99, 102–104].

Instrumental Assessments

Oropharyngeal Dysphagia

While the CDE is effective for describing the oral preparatory phase of swallowing, including deficiencies in eating skills and for behaviors associated with eating [96], it has limitations for discriminating events in the oropharyngeal and esophageal phases of swallowing. DeMatteo and colleagues tested these limitations and found that experienced clinicians could detect aspiration of fluids with a sensitivity of 92 % in the CDE as compared to the videofluoroscopic swallowing study (VFSS). Sensitivity for aspiration of solid food, however, was less adequate at 33 %. Sensitivity for esophageal disorder was not tested.

Instrumental assessments are indicated when it is expected that the results will further describe the parameters of the disorder and will inform intervention decisions. Typically, clinicians have depended on instrumental measures to supplement the CDE when there are indications that oropharyngeal or esophageal dysphagia involvement is contributing to the disorder or when CDE findings do not adequately explain the symptomatology [105]. The choice of test depends on the presenting signs and symptoms. Videofluoroscopy and fiberoptic endoscopy are well-accepted options in pediatric practice for viewing upper airway and pharyngeal anatomy and bolus motility in the oral and pharyngeal phases of swallowing [92, 106, 107]. In addition, VFSS is indicated for direct viewing of the pharyngeal swallow and screening bolus motility and anatomy in the esophagus [106, 107].

Referral criteria for VFSS or FEES are signs of oropharyngeal dysphagia, a diagnosis that suggests a high prevalence of oropharyngeal dysphagia and risk for aspiration, and the probability that the child will tolerate the examination sufficiently to provide valid results [84, 92, 107–109].

The VFSS is a radiographic, qualitative, dynamic assessment that continues to be considered as the gold standard in pediatrics for assessing the biomechanics of swallowing and the adequacy of airway protection. The limitations include exposure to ionizing radiation, the need for a time-limited examination, the need for patient cooperation, and the challenging test environment [92, 93, 106, 110]. During VFSS the child is in a position that simulates natural feeding but is constrained by the need for lateral and anterior-posterior fluoroscopic views of the swallow. The unique advantage of VFSS is that the bolus can be followed from the mouth into the stomach, providing radiographic views of anatomy and physiology and of the timing, biomechanics, bolus flow, and effectiveness of the whole swallow for a barium-impregnated bolus of solid and liquid food. Visualization of penetration, aspiration, and esophageal function is possible [see authors' note 2 in Case Study Box].

Fiberoptic endoscopic evaluations of swallow without sensory testing (FEES) and with sensory testing (FEEST) are receiving increasing attention as an alternative to VFSS for evaluating pediatric dysphagia [84, 111–114]. During FEES a soft, flexible nasopharyngoscope is inserted in the nose and positioned between the soft palate and the epiglottis (oropharynx). Oral and pharyngeal anatomy and selective swallowing events can be viewed for saliva and the child's typical solid and liquid food in familiar postural alignments. A blackout of the view occurs during pharyngeal contraction obscuring the pharyngeal biomechanics during the pharyngeal swallowing response. Signs of aspiration and penetration are apparent prior or following the swallow. During FEEST puffs of air delivered to the aryepiglottic folds test the sensory threshold for the laryngeal adductor reflex. The resulting laryngopharyngeal sensory threshold (LPST) has been found to be related to the number of abnormal oropharyngeal swallowing function parameters and prevalence of aspiration tended to increase when LPST was severely impaired [112]; however, research on this method is sparse. FEES and FEEST are preferred for the child who has never fed orally or accepts insufficient food for VFSS. It allows observations for structure, non-swallowing functions of the upper airway, management of saliva accumulations, intactness of sensation, and spontaneous swallowing as it occurs for accumulations of saliva, all without the introduction of food [84].

There have been a number of studies comparing FEES and VFSS. A preliminary study that compared the swallowing in infants and children before and after placement of the endoscope in the upper airway found no change in swallowing outcomes, and simultaneous ratings were in agreement [84, 111, 115]. FEES had advantages for detecting anatomical anomalies in the upper airway [111, 116] and for testing pharyngolaryngeal sensation [112] and has similar results for detection of laryngeal penetration and laryngotracheal aspiration with VFSS [117, 118].

There are less invasive procedures that have also been used for the objective evaluation of pediatric oral preparatory and oropharyngeal swallowing; however, clinical applications have been limited. Electromyography (EMG) was found to provide useful information regarding level of effort in labial, mandibular, and cervical musculature during swallowing in older children with Duchenne muscular dystrophy (DMD). The EMG procedure differentiated the normal control subjects from the DMD subjects and was well tolerated [119]. Furthermore, it identified weakness in masseter muscles in children diagnosed with spastic cerebral palsy as compared to normal control subjects [120]. Ultrasound, another one of the objective, less invasive evaluation procedures, has been found to be uniquely suited for the assessment of infant sucking. It was useful for evaluating sucking in infants with ankyloglossia pre- and post-frenulotomy, for evaluating breastfeeding and for comparing lingual and hyoid movement patterns in a premature infant during nonnutritive and nutritive sucking [59, 121–123]. Although its use has been reported infrequently for older children, it has been found to be useful for differentiating the oral preparatory and oropharyngeal swallowing in disabled children from that of control subjects [123, 124].

Esophageal Dysphagia

The differential diagnosis of esophageal dysphagia in children can be challenging for the swallowing specialist and physician and confusing to parents as it often presents as feeding difficulty with similar behavioral and developmental deficiencies as those seen in oral preparation and oropharyngeal phase dysphagia.

Esophageal dysphagia may result from anatomical anomalies, GER, inflammation, or neurological disorder [125–128]. Congenital and acquired anatomical anomalies in the esophagus and motor dysfunction occur less frequently. Videofluoroscopic studies can screen for anatomic abnormalities, such as webs and strictures; for esophageal motor disorders such as achalasia of the upper and lower sphincters; and for mucosal anomalies [128]. An esophageal screening during a VFSS can provide preliminary information that indicates the need for additional assessments [106]. Esophageal pH and pH impedance monitoring may be useful for diagnosis of GERD in infants and children. Endoscopic and histologic evaluations may be used to differentiate eosinophilic esophagitis from GERD [129, 130]. High-resolution manometry is an available technology for differential diagnosis of esophageal motility disorders in children [131] and for pharyngo-esophageal motility disorders [132]. Combinations of manometry and videofluoroscopy and manometry and impedance techniques have been reported to provide objective measures of pharyngo-esophageal swallowing dynamics with diagnostic utility in pediatrics [133, 134].

The importance of understanding the mechanics of dysfunction is recognized in the assessment of pediatric dysphagia as a precursor to therapy for the associated swallowing and feeding disorders. Further, early recognition of the diseases and disorders is important for preventing associated maladaptive behaviors [132, 135].

Team Approaches to Dysphagia Evaluation

Although dysphagia in children may present as an isolated developmental, behavioral, or medical disorder that can be adequately managed and resolved by a single clinician, the majority of cases present with multisystem disorders that cross boundaries between health-care disciplines [13]. The benefits are apparent of a team approach for efficient, timely, and effective evaluation and management. Apparent, as well, are the monetary and personal costs of delays in diagnoses and management for children with these complex issues [136, 137]. Distinctions are made between multidisciplinary and transdisciplinary (core team) models with the latter including a more closely integrated collaboration between the involved professionals [138]. Hybrid models include a core transdisciplinary team with interdisciplinary members available on referral. These models have been described as successful for evaluation and differential diagnosis in pediatric dysphagia [1, 13, 84, 139–142]. Team members vary by resources and the needs of the patient population. The composition of a core team may include a medical specialist (e.g., developmental pediatrician or gastroenterologist), speech-language pathology dysphagia specialist, dietician, motor specialist (e.g., occupational or physical therapist), behavioral specialist (e.g., psychologist or behavioral analyst), and family counselor (nurse or social worker). In addition, pediatric medical specialists are consulted on referral for pulmonology, gastroenterology, neurology, otolaryngology, dentistry and dental prosthetics, and surgical specialists.

Treatment in Pediatric Dysphagia

Pediatric intervention includes both daily management and therapy for ingesting solid and liquid foods, ingesting oral medications, and saliva control. Daily management plans are individualized to assure that age-appropriate needs are provided for nutrition, hydration, and airway protection and to maximize quality of life for the child and the family. Therapeutic interventions are selected to advance development of milestone eating skills and behaviors, improve efficiency of eating to support current nutritional demands and growth, and advance skills for swallowing safety [2, 46]. Research has been limited overall. The purpose of this section is to review evidence-based intervention practices and the recent literature.

Treatment Teams

A majority of infants and children with dysphagia have physiological/medical etiologies that occur in combination with behavioral and developmental deficits. The benefits of team management have been apparent in cases that straddle health specialties [7, 13, 136]. A variety of intensive, team-oriented, treatment programs have been found to be effective for treating infants and children in inpatient, outpatient, and school settings [85, 139, 141, 143, 144]. As in evaluation, those children with swallowing and feeding disorder with singular areas of involvement may be managed successfully by an individual specialist. However, team management should be considered when a problem is not resolving as expected.

Compensatory Interventions

Compensatory strategies are generally considered to be those interventions that have been found to support improved swallowing performance, but results do not continue once the strategy is withdrawn [145]. However, in pediatric dysphagia, compensatory strategies may be used to support practice in less mature and less demanding eating tasks in infants and children for whom the practice is intended to improve skill. In those cases, the strategies are, arguably, therapeutic – which is used to make durable changes in function.

Positioning

The effect of postural alignment and seating supports is generally acknowledged to be important in all stages of development for eating skills [146–148]. Larnet and Ekberg (1995) observed reductions in aspiration and posterior oral leakage of the bolus when children with cerebral palsy (CP) were supported with head-neck flexion as compared to extension [147]. Special considerations for seating for VFSS studies and the implications for making recommendations for eating were discussed by Arvedson and Lefton-Greif [92].

Studies of positioning effects on feeding in the neonate have found more significant differences earlier in the transition from tube to oral feeds than later in the transition. A semi-elevated side-lying position during bottle-feeding resulted in better regulation of breathing and heart rate stability for very preterm infants [149]. Sick neonates were found to have more favorable oxygen saturation, larger tidal volume, and more favorable sucking parameters in prone position as compared to supine position [150]. However, little difference was found in a cohort of older premature infants when fed in side-lying or cradle-hold position [151]. The complex effects of positioning in premature infants are illustrated by Omari and colleagues (2004) who demonstrated significantly different effects of the right and left lateral position on frequency of transient lower esophageal relaxation and associated gastroesophageal reflux in healthy infants at 35–37 weeks postmenstrual age [152].

Food Viscosity and Texture

In pediatric practice, solid food viscosity, tastes and texture, and liquid viscosity and tastes are manipulated as compensation for functional deficiencies and as therapeutic strategies for advancing sensory tolerances and developmental skills. Some of these practices are empirical rather than evidence based. Foods may be thickened as compensation to increase ease of containing the bolus in the mouth and controlling the bolus for initiation and completion of the swallow. Or they may be thinned for ease of oral transport and pharyngeal clearance. Tastes and textures are manipulated for preference and for promptness of swallow initiation. When used as therapeutic strategies, these features are manipulated to train functional skills for milestones, such as chewing or drinking from a cup or to improve coordinations for the oral preparation phase of swallowing. In pediatric practice, bolus characteristics are often modified with food additives rather than commercial thickening agents, although pre-thickened liquids may be used [153]. The advisability of using commercial thickeners and other thickening agents as a swallowing compensation in bottle-feeding has been questioned [154], and clinicians are cautioned to collaborate with dieticians for use of this strategy with premature and young infants.

Specialized Equipment for Feeding
Decisions regarding the use of specialized equipment during feeding are largely empirical. Feeding equipment to support swallowing may include positioning equipment for adaptive positions for eating [85, 145]. Specialized spoons, cups, and straws may be used to facilitate oral management of the bolus and to regulate bolus size. Studies have explored the effect of nipple selection on feeding [155] and the usefulness of nipple accessories for breastfeeding [156] in premature and very-low-birth-weight infants.

Rehabilitative Interventions

Selection of therapeutic swallowing and feeding interventions depends on contributing causes as well as on the child's dysphagia profile. Optimally, contributing medical, structural, and environmental conditions are resolved or mitigated through medical or surgical treatments and family education so as to support the child in rehabilitation [13]. Behavior modification strategies address behavioral problems that affect motivation for eating and eating pragmatics. Functional practice strategies address training for the advancing developmental skills. The two areas of disorder, behaviors and skills, have been referred to as "sensory-based" and "motor-based" functions to distinguish the issues that respond to behavior modification-based strategies (often seen as grounded in sensory processing deficiencies and sensory aversions) from issues that respond to functional practice (generally seen as grounded in neuromotor deficiencies and deprivation of appropriate and sufficient practice) [1]. However, in those children where both behavioral and skill deficiencies are seen, treating these aspects as an integrated problem provides optimum outcomes for health, functional skill, and social participation [see authors' note 3 in Case Study Box].

The primary concerns for nutrition and respiratory health are limiting factors in pediatric rehabilitation. It is crucial that treatments to advance skills and improve behaviors do not interfere with the child's ability to maintain growth or jeopardize airway protection. These concerns guide selection of strategies, the rate of change in program goals and objectives, and the ultimate goals for outcomes of the program.

Pediatric Habilitation and Rehabilitation

Pediatric dysphagia treatment involves managing the child's current needs for airway protection, nutrition and hydration, maintaining optimum eating behaviors and skills, and advancing behaviors and skills to meet the nutritional, developmental, and social needs of the growing child [64]. When these needs cannot be met by oral feeding, tube feeding may be used to supplement or substitute for oral feeding [5, 13, 157]. This occurs typically in the very-low-birth-weight and premature infant [158]. Tube feeding can be initiated as well in the older child who may fail to thrive as demands for nutritional intake increase or is unable to protect their airway during eating [159, 160]. However, difficulties with swallowing and feeding often occur when tube feeding is no longer needed and demands are made for making the transition from tube to oral feeding [161, 162].

For the oral feeding, child with dysphagia and related feeding disorder treatment goals include advancing their skills for managing puree and solid foods, for chewing, biting, drinking from a cup and straw, and feeding themselves. For the child with behavioral involvements, goals are included for gaining and maintaining the appropriate motivations for eating, for managing the eating pragmatics that are the social-interactive aspects of eating, and for the acceptance of a nutritionally acceptable variety of foods [2, 46]. Furthermore, in those children with chronic dysphagia, treatment includes the ongoing refinement of swallowing and feeding efficiency that is needed to maintain growth and hydration into adulthood [46]. Therapeutic interventions are needed as well in those children for whom saliva swallowing and saliva control are deficient [20, 163, 164] and those who have not acquired the needed skills and behaviors for swallowing medications [165].

Therapeutic Strategies

Transition from Tube to Oral Feeding

Facilitating the transition from tube to oral feeding in the infant and advancing sucking skills are the primary goals of dysphagia management in the Neonatal Intensive Care Unit (NICU) [85, 166]. Evidence is available on effectiveness of oral stimulation routines [167], nonnutritive sucking [168, 169], and external pacing [170] among other strategies for facilitating the transition [20]. For infants who do not make a successful transition to oral feeding and for those whom tube feeding is initiated later in childhood, feeding and swallowing difficulties occur and require remediation [105, 161, 162]. These children often require team approaches for developing and implementing programs for the behavioral, developmental, and neuromotor problems that are interfering with their transition to oral feeding [141, 144, 171] and subsequent acquisition of mature swallowing and feeding skills and behaviors [20, 144, 172].

Behavioral Modification Strategies

There has been considerable research on strategies for improving motivation for eating, acceptance of food variety, and the cooperative pragmatics for eating [31, 173]. These strategies have been found to be successful in reducing food refusal, facilitating participation in eating exercises and meals, increasing the swallowing of food, and supporting independence for eating [20, 174].

Motor Learning for Functional Skills

Motor learning strategies refer to a variety of approaches for structuring exercises. They are implemented in order to optimize the effects of the practice for acquisition and improvement of motor skills and retention of treatment effects [20, 172]. These strategies may be used in conjunction with *consistent functional practice* [175] and multicomponent treatments such as *oral sensory-motor therapy* [20, 144, 176, 177] as well as behavioral strategies to enhance treatment effects. Children with neuromuscular disorders such as cerebral palsy have been found to benefit from motor-based treatments and compensations [178, 179]; however, their risk for nutritional failure and aspiration warrants careful consideration when training advanced eating skills [105].

Long-Term Outcomes

We have few studies of long-term outcomes of treatment for children with feeding disorders. In a cohort of children 1 month to 10 years old, 5-year outcomes for improvement in swallowing function were found to be variable depending on presenting symptoms. Children with neurologic conditions showed less favorable outcomes as compared to those with non-neurologic etiologies [180]. However, overall significant favorable changes did occur in both groups. In a 3-year study of cost-effectiveness of treatment, children attending a multidisciplinary team feeding clinic were found to improve in their swallowing and feeding disorder and to have reduced frequency of doctor visits [181].

Summary

In summary, dysphagia in children is a complex disorder, often involving behavioral, physiologic, and developmental features. Typically the onset is in infancy. The dysphagia may resolve or persist into adulthood as a chronic disorder. Treatment approaches may utilize a team of interventionists to manage multiple system involvement or individual clinicians in some instances. In order to optimize respiratory health, nutrition, behaviors, and functional skill in the short and long term, the treatment program includes daily management of eating, drinking, and taking oral medications and therapy. Treatment approaches include behavioral strategies and functional practice augmented by the use of evidence-based motor learning strategies and sensory-motor exercise. Functional improvements in swallowing and feeding are seen to result from evidence-based interventions; however, research is needed to further explore long-term outcomes.

References

1. Arvedson JC. Assessment of pediatric dysphagia and feeding disorders: clinical and instrumental approaches. Dev Disabil Res Rev. 2008;14:118–27.
2. Sheppard JJ. Clinical evaluation and treatment. In: Rosenthal SR, Sheppard JJ, Lotze M, editors. Dysphagia and the child with developmental disabilities. San Diego: Singular Publishing Group; 1994. p. 37–75.
3. Fung E, Samson-Fang L, Stallings VA, Conaway M, Liptak G, Henderson RC, et al. Feeding dysfunction is associated with poor growth and health status in children with cerebral palsy. J Am Diet Assoc. 2002;102(3):361–73.
4. Stevenson RD, Haves RP, Cater LV, Blackman JA. Clinical correlates of linear growth in children with cerebral palsy. Dev Med Child Neurol. 1994;36(2):135–42.
5. Calis E, Veugelers R, Sheppard JJ, Tibboel D, Evenhuis H, Penning C. Dysphagia in children with severe generalized cerebral palsy and intellectual disability. Dev Med Child Neurol. 2008;50(8):625–30.
6. Wilson E, Hustad KC. Early feeding abilities in children with cerebral palsy: a parent report study. J Med Speech Lang Pathol. 2009;17:31–44.
7. Burklow K, Phelps A, Schultz J, McConnell K, Rudolph C. Classifying complex pediatric feeding disorders. J Pediatr Gastroenterol Nutr. 1998;27(2):143–7.
8. Lefton-Greif M, Arvedson J. Pediatric feeding and swallowing disorders: state of health, population trends, and application of the international classification of functioning, disability, and health. Semin Speech Lang. 2007;28(3):161–5.
9. Linscheid T. Behavioral treatments for pediatric feeding disorders. Behav Modif. 2006;30(1):6–23.
10. Nadon G, Feldman D, Gisel E. Feeding issues associated with autism spectrum disorders. In: Fitzgerald M, editor. Recent advances in autism spectrum disorders, vol. 1. Rijeka: InTech; 2013. p. 559–632.
11. Parkes J, Hill N, Platt M, Donnelly C. Oromotor dysfunction and communication impairments in children with cerebral palsy: a register study. Dev Med Child Neurol. 2010;52(12):1113–9.
12. Reilly S, Skuse D, Poblete X. Prevalence of feeding problems and oral motor dysfunction in children with cerebral palsy: a community survey. J Pediatr. 1996;129(6):877–82.
13. Rommel N, De Meyer AM, Feenstra L, Veereman-Wauters G. The complexity of feeding problems in 700 infants and young children presenting to a tertiary care institution. J Pediatr Gastroenterol Nutr. 2003;37:75–82.
14. Roden DF, Altman KW. Causes of dysphagia among different age groups: a systematic review of the literature. Otolaryngol Clin North Am. 2013;46(6):965–87.
15. Dodrill P. Feeding difficulties in preterm infants. ICAN Infant Child Adolesc Nutr. 2011;3(6):324–31.
16. Da Costa SP, Van der Schans CP, Zweens MJ, Boelema SR, Van der Meij E, Boerman MA, et al. The development of sucking patterns in preterm, small-for-gestational age infants. J Pediatr. 2010;157(4):603–9.
17. Medoff-Cooper B, McGrath JM, Bilker W. Nutritive sucking and neurobehavioral development in preterm infants from 34 weeks PCA to term. MCN Am J Matern Child Nurs. 2000;25(2):64–70.

18. Lau C, Smith EO, Schanler RJ. Coordination of suck-swallow and swallow respiration in preterm infants. Acta Paediatr. 2003;92(6):721–7.
19. O'Neill AC, Richter GT. Pharyngeal dysphagia in children with Down syndrome. Otolaryngol Head Neck Surg. 2013;149(1):146–50.
20. Sheppard J. Management of oral pharyngeal dysphagia in pediatrics: rehabilitative maneuvers and exercise. In: Shaker R, Easterling C, Belafsky PC, Postma GN, editors. Manual of diagnostic and therapeutic techniques for disorders of deglutition. New York: Springer; 2013. p. 319–48.
21. Morgan AT, Mageandran SD, Mei C. Incidence and clinical presentation of dysarthria and dysphagia in the acute setting following paediatric traumatic brain injury. Child Care Health Dev. 2010;36(1):44–53.
22. Pollack IF, Polinko P, Albright AL, Towbin R, Fitz C. Mutism and pseudobulbar symptoms after resection of posterior fossa tumors in children: incidence and pathophysiology. Neurosurgery. 1995;37(5):885–93.
23. Buckley RT, Morgan T, Saneto RP, Barber J, Ellenbogen RG, Ojemann JG. Dysphagia after pediatric functional hemispherectomy. J Neurosurg Pediatr. 2014;13(1):95–100.
24. Robbins J, Daniels S, Baredes S. Diagnostic-based treatment approaches. In: Blitzer MB, Ramig L, editors. Neurologic disorders of the larynx. 2nd ed. New York: Thieme; 2009. p. 149–59.
25. Malandraki GA, Sutton BP, Perlman AL, Karampinos DC, Conway C. Neural activation of swallowing and swallowing-related tasks in healthy young adults: an attempt to separate the components of deglutition. Hum Brain Mapp. 2009;30(10):3209–26.
26. Cooper-Brown L, Copeland S, Dailey S, Downey D, Petersen MC, Stimson C, et al. Feeding and swallowing dysfunction in genetic syndromes. Dev Disabil Res Rev. 2008;14(2):147–57.
27. Miller CK. Feeding issues and interventions in infants and children with clefts and craniofacial syndromes. Semin Speech Lang. 2011;32(2):115–26.
28. Romano AA, Allanson JE, Dahlgren J, Gelb BD, Hall B, Pierpont ME, et al. Noonan syndrome: clinical features, diagnosis, and management guidelines. Pediatrics. 2010;126(4):746–59.
29. Georgia A. Malandraki, Melissa Roth, Justine Joan Sheppard. Telepractice for Pediatric Dysphagia: A Case Study. International Journal of Telerehabilitation. 2014;6(1):3–16
30. Tuchman D, Walter R. Disorders of feeding and swallowing in infants and children: pathophysiology, diagnosis, and treatment. San Diego: Singular Publishing Group; 1994.
31. Patel M. Assessment of pediatric feeding disorders. In: Reed DD, DiGennaro R, Florence D, Luiselli JK, editors. Handbook of crisis intervention and developmental disabilities. New York: Springer; 2013. p. 169–82.
32. Kumar V, Mathai SS, Kanitkar M. Preliminary study in to the incidence of gastroesophageal reflux (GER) in high risk neonates admitted to NICU. Indian J Pediatr. 2012;79(9):1197–200.
33. Czinn SJ, Blanchard S. Gastroesophageal reflux disease in neonates and infants: when and how to treat. Paediatr Drugs. 2013;15(1):19–27.
34. Hyman PE. Gastroesophageal reflux: one reason why baby won't eat. J Pediatr. 1994;125(6): S103–9.
35. Fishman LB, Bousvaros A. Gastrointestinal issues. In: Rubin IL, Crocker AC, editors. Medical care for children & adults with developmental disabilities. 2nd ed. Baltimore: Paul H. Brookes Pub; 2006. p. 113–9.
36. Gupte AR, Draganov PV. Eosinophilic esophagitis. World J Gastroenterol. 2009;15(1):17–24.
37. Sorser SA, Barawi M, Hagglund K, Almojaned M, Lyons H. Eosinophilic esophagitis in children and adolescents: epidemiology, clinical presentation and seasonal variation. J Gastroenterol. 2013;48(1):81–5.
38. Noel RJ, Putnam PE, Rothenberg ME. Eosinophilic esophagitis. N Engl J Med. 2004;351(9):940–1.
39. Di Scipio WJ, Kaslon K. Conditioned dysphagia in cleft palate children after pharyngeal flap surgery. Psychosom Med. 1982;44(3):247–57.
40. Miller CK, Linck J, Willging JP. Duration and extent of dysphagia following pediatric airway reconstruction. Int J Pediatr Otorhinolaryngol. 2009;73(4):573–9.

41. Norman V, Louw B, Kritzinger A. Incidence and description of dysphagia in infants and toddlers with tracheostomies: a retrospective review. Int Pediatr Otorhinolaryngol. 2007;71(7):1087–92.
42. Schreck KA, Williams K, Smith AF. A comparison of eating behaviors between children with and without autism. J Autism Dev Disord. 2004;34(4):433–8.
43. Williams PG, Dalrymple N, Neal J. Eating habits of children with autism. Pediatr Nurs. 2000;26(3):259–64.
44. Williams K, Seiverling L. Eating problems in children with Autism Spectrum Disorders. Top Clin Nutr. 2010;25(1):27–37.
45. Raiten DJ, Massaro T. Perspectives on the nutritional ecology of autistic children. J Autism Dev Disord. 1986;16(2):133–43.
46. Sheppard JJ. Intellectual and developmental disability. In: Jones H, Rosenbek J, editors. Dysphagia in rare conditions, an encyclopedia. San Diego: Plural Publishing; 2010.
47. Patel M, Piazza C, Kelly M, Ochsner C, Santana C. Using a fading procedure to increase fluid consumption in a child with feeding problems. J Appl Behav Anal. 2001;34:357–60.
48. Twachtman-Reilly J, Amaral SC, Zebrowski PP. Addressing feeding disorders in children on the autism spectrum in school-based settings: physiological and behavioral issues. Lang Speech Hear Serv Sch. 2008;39(2):261–72.
49. Larsen WJ. Essentials of human embryology. New York: Churchill Livingstone; 1998.
50. Moore KL, Hay JC. The developing human; clinically oriented embryology. Philadelphia: Saunders; 1973.
51. Bush JO, Jiang R. Palatogenesis: morphogenetic and molecular mechanisms of secondary palate development. Development. 2012;139(2):231–43.
52. Kuo B, Urma D. Esophagus–anatomy and development. GI Motil Online. 2006.
53. Bradley RM, Stern IB. The development of the human taste bud during the foetal period. J Anat. 1967;101(4):743–52.
54. Kurjak A, Azumendi G, Vecek N, Kupesic S, Solak M, Varga D, et al. Fetal hand movements and facial expression in normal pregnancy studied by four-dimensional sonography. J Perinat Med. 2003;31(6):496–508.
55. Miller J, Cheng J, Macedonia C. A three-dimensional examination of aerodigestive development in the living, human fetus: prenatal perspectives on emerging oral, digestive and respiratory function. Dysphagia. 2005;20(10).
56. Miller JL, Sonies BC, Macedonia C. Emergence of oropharyngeal, laryngeal and swallowing activity in the developing fetal upper aerodigestive tract: an ultrasound evaluation. Early Hum Dev. 2003;71(1):61–87.
57. Ross MG, Nijland MJ. Development of ingestive behavior. Am J Physiol. 1998;274(4):879–93.
58. Petrikovsky B, Kaplan G, Pestrak H. The application of color Doppler technology to the study of fetal swallowing. Obst Gynaecol. 1995;86:605–8.
59. Miller J, Kang S. Preliminary ultrasound observation of lingual movement patterns during nutritive versus non-nutritive sucking in a premature infant. Dysphagia. 2007;22:150–60.
60. Mistretta CM, Bradley RM. Taste and swallowing in utero. Br Med Bull. 1975;31(1):80–4.
61. Liley AW. Pathophysiology of gestation. In: Assali NS, ABrinkman CR, editors. Pathophysiology of gestation. New York: Academic; 1972. p. 157–206.
62. Arvedson JC. Swallowing and feeding in infants and young children. PART 1 Oral cavity, pharynx and esophagus. GI Motility online 2006. doi:10.1038/gimo17, Published 16 May 2006
63. Logemann JA. Oropharyngeal dysphagia and nutritional management. Curr Opin Clin Nutr Metab Care. 2007;10(5):611–4.
64. Delaney AL, Arvedson JC. Development of swallowing and feeding: prenatal through first year of life. Dev Disabil Res Rev. 2008;14(2):105–17.
65. Kelly BN, Huckabee ML, Jones RD, Frampton CM. The early impact of feeding on infant breathing-swallowing coordination. Respir Physiol Neurobiol. 2007;156(2):147–53.
66. Jacobs LA, Dickinson JE, Hart PD, Doherty DA, Faulkner SJ. Normal nipple position in term infants measured on breastfeeding ultrasound. J Hum Lact. 2007;23(1):52–9.
67. Chey WY, Lee KY. Motilin. Clin Gastroenterol. 1980;9(3):645–56.

68. Kimble C. Nonnutritive sucking: adaptation and health for the neonate. Neonatal Netw. 1992;11(2):29–33.
69. Lau C, Alagugurusamy R, Schanler RJ, Smith EO, Shulman RJ. Characterization of the developmental stages of sucking in preterm infants during bottle feeding. Acta Paediatr. 2000;89(7):846–52.
70. Landy S. Pathways to competence: encouraging healthy social and emotional development in young children. 2nd ed. Baltimore: Paul H. Brookes Pub; 2009.
71. Folio MR. PDMS-2: peabody developmental motor scales. 2nd ed. Austin: Pro-Ed; 2000.
72. Piper MC, Darrah J. Motor assessment of the developing infant. Philadelphia: Saunders; 1994.
73. Carruth BR, Skinner JD. Feeding behaviors and other motor development in healthy children (2–24 months). J Am Coll Nutr. 2002;21(2):88–96.
74. Rossetti L. The Rossetti infant-toddler language scale: a measure of communication and interaction. East Moline: LinguiSystems Inc; 1990.
75. Northstone K, Emmett P, Nethersole F. The effect of age of introduction to lumpy solids on foods eaten and reported feeding difficulties at 6 and 15 months. J Hum Nutr Diet. 2001;14(1):43–54.
76. Green J, Moore C, Ruark J. Development of chewing in children from 12 to 48 months: longitudinal study of EMG patterns. J Neurophysiol. 1997;77:2704–16.
77. Gisel EG. Effect of food texture on the development of chewing of children between six months and two years of age. Dev Med Child Neurol. 1991;33(1):69–79.
78. Sheppard J. Using motor learning approaches for treating swallowing and feeding disorders: a review. Lang Speech Hear Serv Schools. 2008;39(2):227–36.
79. Illingworth R, Lister J. The critical or sensitive period with special reference to certain feeding problems in infants and children. J Pediatr. 1964;65:840–8.
80. Hensch TK. Critical period plasticity in local cortical circuits. Nat Rev Neurosci. 2005;6:877–88.
81. Coulthard H, Harris G, Emmett P. Delayed introduction of lumpy foods to children during the complementary feeding period affects child's food acceptance and feeding at 7 years of age. Matern Child Nutr. 2009;5(1):75–85.
82. Cashdan E. A sensitive period for learning about food. Hum Nature. 1994;5(3):279–91.
83. Morgan A, Reilly S. Clinical signs, aetiologies and characteristics of paediatric dysphagia. In: Cichero J, Murdoch B, editors. Dysphagia, foundation, theory and practice. New York: Wiley; 2006. p. 391–465.
84. Willging JP, Miller CK, Link DT, Rudolph CD. Use of FEES to assess and manage pediatric patients. In: Langmore SE, editor. Endoscopic evaluation and treatment of dysphagia. New York: Thieme; 2001. p. 213–34.
85. Sheppard JJ, Fletcher KR. Evidence-based interventions for breast and bottle feeding in the neonatal intensive care unit. Semin Speech Lang. 2007;28:204–12.
86. Suiter DM, Leder SB, Karas DE. The 3-ounce (90-cc) water swallow challenge: a screening test for children with suspected oropharyngeal dysphagia. Otolaryngol Head Neck Surg. 2009;140:187–90.
87. Sheppard JJ, Hochman R, Baer C. The dysphagia disorder survey: validation of an assessment for swallowing and feeding function in developmental disability. Res Dev Disabil. 2014;35(5):929–42.
88. Lukens CT, Linscheid TR. Development and validation of an inventory to assess mealtime behavior problems in children with autism. J Autism Dev Disord. 2008;38(2):342–52.
89. Crist W, Dobbelsteyn C, Brousseau AM, Napier-Phillips A. Pediatric assessment scale for severe feeding problems: validity and reliability of a new scale for tube-fed children. Nutr Clin Pract. 2004;19:403–8.
90. Thoyre SM, Pados BF, Park J, Estrem H, Hodges EA, McComish C, et al. Development and content validation of the Pediatric Eating Assessment Tool (Pedi-EAT). Am J Speech Lang Pathol. 2014;23:46–59.

91. Hendy HM, Williams KE, Camise TS, Eckman N, Hedemann A. The Parent Mealtime Action Scale (PMAS). Development and association with children's diet and weight. Appetite. 2009;52:328–39.
92. Arvedson JC, Lefton-Greif MA. Pediatric videofluoroscopic swallow studies: a professional manual with caregiver guidelines. San Antonia: Communication Skill Builders; 1998.
93. Rommel N. Assessment techniques for babies, infants and children. In: Cichero J, Murdoch B, editors. Dysphagia, foundation, theory and practice. New York: Wiley; 2006. p. 466–86.
94. Pitcher J, Crandall M, Goodrich SJ. Pediatric clinical feeding assessment. In: Rebecca L, Kendall K, editors. Dysphagia assessment and treatment planning: a team approach. San Diego: Plural Publishing; 2008. p. 117–36.
95. Howe T, Lin K, Fu C, Sa C, Hsieh C. A review of psychometric properties of feeding assessment tools used in neonates. J Obstet Gynecol Neonatal Nurs. 2008;37(3):338–49.
96. Benfer KA, Weir KA, Boyd RN. Clinimetrics of measures of oropharyngeal dysphagia for preschool children with cerebral palsy and neurodevelopmental disabilities: a systematic review. Dev Med Child Neurol. 2012;54:784–95.
97. Bingham PM, Ashikaga T, Abbasi S. Relationship of Neonatal Oral Motor Assessment Scale to feeding performance of premature infants. J Neonatal Nurs. 2012;18:30–6.
98. Zarem C, Kidokoro H, Neil J, Wallendorf M, Inder T, Pineda R. Psychometrics of the neonatal oral motor assessment scale. Dev Med Child Neurol. 2013;55:1115–20.
99. Remijn L, Speyer R, Groen BE, Holtus PC, van Limbeek J, Nijhuis-van der Sanden MW. Assessment of mastication in healthy children and children with cerebral palsy: a validity and consistency study. J Oral Rehabil. 2013;40(5):336–47.
100. Sellers D, Mandy A, Pennington L, Hankins M, Morris C. Development and reliability of a system to classify the eating and drinking ability of people with cerebral palsy. Dev Med Child Neurol. 2013;56(3):245–51.
101. Sellers D, Pennington L, Mandy A, Morris C. A systematic review of ordinal scales used to classify the eating and drinking abilities of individuals with cerebral palsy. Dev Med Child Neurol. 2013;56(4):313–22.
102. Reid SM, Johnson HM, Reddihough DS. The Drooling Impact Scale: a measure of the impact of drooling in children with developmental disabilities. Dev Med Child Neurol. 2010;52:e23–8.
103. Chatoor I, Getson P, Menvielle E, Brassearx C, O'Donnell R, Rivera Y, et al. A feeding scale for research and clinical practice to assess mother-infant interactions in the first three years of life. Inf Mental Hlth J. 1997;18(1):76–91.
104. Williams KE, Hendy HM, Seiverling LJ, Can SH. Validation of the parent mealtime action scale (PMAS) when applied to children referred to a hospital-based feeding clinic. Appetite. 2011;56(3):553–7.
105. Arvedson JC. Feeding children with cerebral palsy and swallowing difficulties. Eur J Clin Nutr. 2013;67:S9–12.
106. Marquis J, Pressman H. Radiologic assessment of pediatric swallowing. In: Rosenthal SR, Sheppard JJ, Lotze M, editors. Dysphagia and the child with developmental disabilities, medical, clinical and family interventions. San Diego: Singular Publishing Group; 1994. p. 189–207.
107. Easterling C. Food for thought: the esophagus, to screen or not to screen…that is the question, the responsibility, and liability. Perspect Swallow Swallow Disord (Dysphagia). 2012;21(2):68–72.
108. Lefton-Greif MA, McGrath-Morrow SA. Deglutition and respiration: development, coordination, and practical implications. Semin Speech Lang. 2007;28(3):166–79.
109. Cass H, Wallis C, Ryan MM, Reilly S, McHugh K. Assessing pulmonary consequences of dysphagia in children with neurological disabilities: when to intervene? Dev Med Child Neurol. 2005;47:347–52.
110. Hiorns MP, Ryan MM. Current practice in paediatric videofluoroscopy. Pediatr Radiol. 2006;36:911–9.

111. Boseley ME, Ashland J, Hartnick CJ. The utility of the fiberoptic endoscopic evaluation of swallowing (FEES) in diagnosing and treating children with Type I laryngeal clefts. Int J Pediatr Otorhinolaryngol. 2006;70:339–43.
112. Ulualp S, Brown A, Sanghavi R, Rivera-Sanchez Y. Assessment of laryngopharyngeal sensation in children with dysphagia. Laryngoscope. 2013;123:2291–5.
113. Sitton M, Arvedson JC, Visotcky A, Braun N, Kerschner J, Tarima S, et al. Fiberoptic Endoscopic Evaluation of Swallowing in children: feeding outcomes related to diagnostic groups and endoscopic findings. Int J Pediatr Otorhinolaryngol. 2011;75:1024–31.
114. Boesch RP, Daines C, Willging JP, Kaul A, Cohen AP, Wood RE, et al. Advances in the diagnosis and management of chronic pulmonary aspiration in children. Eur Respir J. 2006;28:847–61.
115. Willging JP, Miller CK, McConnell K, Rudolph C. Lack of effect of fiberoptic endoscope passage on swallowing function in children. Dysphagia. 1997;12:131.
116. Miller CK, Willging JP, Strife JL, Rudolph CD. Fiberoptic endoscope examination of swallowing in infants and children with feeding disorders. Dysphagia. 1994;9:266.
117. DaSilva AP, Lubianca Neto JF, Lantoro PP. Comparison between videofluoroscopy and endoscopic evaluation of swallowing for the diagnosis of dysphagia in children. Otolaryngol Head Neck Surg. 2010;143:204–9.
118. Leder SB, Karas DE. Fiberoptic endoscopic evaluation of swallowing in the pediatric population. Laryngoscope. 2000;110(7):1132–2000.
119. Archer SK, Garrod R, Hart N, Miller S. Dysphagia in Duchenne muscular dystrophy assessed objectively by surface electromyography. Dysphagia. 2013;28:188–98.
120. Santos MT, Manzano FS, Chamlian TR, Masiero D, Jardim JR. Effect of spastic cerebral palsy on jaw-closing muscles during clenching. Spec Care Dentist. 2010;30(4):163–7.
121. Geddes DT, Chadwick CP, Kent JC, Garbin CP, Hartmann PE. Ultrasound imaging of infant swallowing during breast-feeding. Dysphagia. 2010;25:183–91.
122. Geddes DT, Langton DB, Gollow I, Jacobs LA, Hartmann PE, Simmer K. Frenulotomy for breastfeeding infants with ankyloglossia: effect on milk removal and sucking mechanism as imaged by ultrasound. Pediatrics. 2008;122(1):e188–94.
123. Yang WT, Loveday EJ, Metreweli C, Sullivan PB. Ultrasound assessment of swallowing in malnourished disabled children. Br J Radiol. 1997;70(838):992–4.
124. Casas MJ, McPherson KA, Kenny DJ. Durational aspects of oral swallow in neurologically normal children and children with cerebral palsy: an ultrasound investigation. Dysphagia. 1995;10:155–9.
125. Mukkada VA, Haas A, Maune NC, Capocelli KE, Henry M, Gilman N, et al. Feeding dysfunction in children with eosinophilic gastrointestinal diseases. Pediatrics. 2010;126(3):e672–7.
126. Weir KA, McMahon S, Taylor S, Chang AB. Oropharyngeal aspiration and silent aspiration in children. Chest. 2011;140(3):589–97.
127. Yellen RF, Goldberg H. Update on gastroesophageal reflux disease in pediatric airway disorders. Am J Med. 2001;111(8):1.
128. Tipnes NA. Special consideration in the evaluation of infants with deglultitive disorders. In: Shaker R, Easterling C, Belafsky PC, Postma GN, editors. Manual of diagnostic and therapeutic techniques for disorders of deglutition. New York: Springer; 2013. p. 389–95.
129. Vendenplas Y, Rudolph CD, DiLorenzo C, Hassall E, Liptak G, Mazur L, et al. Pediatric gastroesophageal reflux clinical practice guidelines: joint recommendations of the North American Society for Pediatric Gastroenerology, Hepatology and Nutrition (NASPGHAN) and European Society for Pediatric Gastroenterology, Hepatology, and Nutrition (ESPGHAN). J Pediatr Gastroenterol Nutr. 2009;40(4):498–547.
130. Chan CY, Jadcherla SR. Clinical perspectives in esophageal disorders in infants. ASHA Lead. 2012;21(2). doi: 10.1044/sasd21.2.52
131. Goldani HA, Staiano A, Borrelli O, Thapar N, Lindley KJ. Pediatric esophageal high-resolution manometry: utility of a standardized protocol and size-adjusted pressure topography parameters. Am J Gastroenterol. 2010;105:460–7.

132. Rommel N, Omari T. Abnormal pharyngoesophageal function in infants and young children: diagnosis with high-resolution manometry. J Pediatr Gastroenterol Nutr. 2011;52 Suppl 1:S29–30.
133. Rommel N, Dejaeger E, Bellon E, Smet M, Veereman-Wauters G. Videomanometry reveals clinically relevant parameters of swallowing in children. Int J Pediatr Otorhinolaryngol. 2006;70:1397–405.
134. Omari T, Dejaeger E, Van Beckevoort D, Goeleven A, De Cock P, Hoffman I, et al. A novel method for the nonradiological assessment of ineffective swallowing. Am J Gastroenterol. 2011;106:1796–802.
135. Rosen JM, Lavenbarg T, Cocjin J, Hyman PE. Diffuse esophageal spasm in children referred for manometry. J Pediatr Gastroenterol Nutr. 2013;56:436–8.
136. Reilly S, Carr L. Foreign body ingestion in children with severe developmental disability: a case study. Dysphagia. 2001;16:68–73.
137. Sheppard JJ. Editorial case management challenges in pediatric dysphagia. Dysphagia. 2001;16:74.
138. Rosen C, Miller C, Pitten IM, Bicchieri S, Gordon RM, Daniele R. Team approaches to treating children with disabilities: a comparison. Arch Phys Med Rehabil. 1998;79:430–4.
139. Miller CK, Burklow KA, Santoro K, Kirby E, Mason D, Rudolph C. An interdisciplinary team approach to management of pediatric feeding and swallowing disorders. Child Health Care. 2001;30(3):201–18.
140. Santoro A, Lang MBD, Moretti E, Sellari-Franceschini S, Orazini L, Cipriani P, et al. A proposed multidisciplinary approach for identifying feeding abnormalities in children with cerebral palsy. J Child Neurol. 2012;27(6):708–12.
141. Roche WJ, Eicher PS, Martorana P, Berkowitz M, Petronchak J, Dzioba J, et al. An oral, motor, medical and behavioral approach to pediatric feeding and swallowing disorders: an interdisciplinary model. Perspect Swallow Swallow Disord (Dysphagia). 2011;20:65–74.
142. Bryan D, Pressman H. Comprehensive team evaluation. In: Rosenthal SR, Sheppard JJ, Lotze M, editors. Dysphagia and the child with developmental disabilities, medical, clinical, and family interventions. San Diego: Singular Publishing Group; 1994. p. 15–36.
143. Milnes SM, Piazza CC. Intensive treatment of pediatric feeding disorders. In: Reed DD, Reed FDD, Luiselli JK, editors. Handbook of crisis intervention and developmental disabilities, Issues in clinical child psychology. New York: Springer; 2013. p. 398–408.
144. McKirdy L, Sheppard JJ, Osborne M, Payne P. Transition from tube to oral feeding in the school setting. Lang Speech Hear Serv Sch. 2008;39(1):249–60.
145. Miller CK, Willging JP. Compensatory strategies and techniques. In: Shaker R, Easterling C, Belafsky PC, Postma GN, editors. Manual of diagnostic and therapeutic techniques for disorders of deglutition. New York: Springer; 2013. p. 349–88.
146. Woods EK. The influence of posture and positioning on oral motor development and dysphagia. In: Rosenthal SR, Sheppard JJ, Lotze M, editors. Dysphagia and the child with developmental disabilities, medical, clinical and family interventions. San Diego: Singular Publishing Group; 1994. p. 153–87.
147. Larnet G, Ekberg O. Positioning improves the oral and pharyngeal swallowing function in children with cerebral palsy. Acta Paediatr. 1995;84(6):689–93.
148. Snider L, Majnemer A, Darsaklis V. Feeding interventions for children with cerebral palsy: a review of the evidence. Phys Occup Ther Pediatr. 2011;31(1):58–77.
149. Park J, Thoyre SM, Knafl GJ, Hodges EA, Nix WG. Efficacy of semi elevated side-lying positioning during bottle-feeding of very preterm infants: a pilot study. J Perinat Neonatal Nurs. 2014;28(1):69–79.
150. Mizuno K, Inoue M, Takeuchi T. The effects of body positioning on sucking behaviour in sick neonates. Eur J Pediatr. 2000;159(11):827–31.
151. Dawson JA, Myers LR, Moorhead A, Jacobs SE, Ong K, Salo F, et al. A randomised trial of two techniques for bottle feeding preterm infants. J Paediatr Child Health. 2013;49(6):462–6.

152. Omari T, Rommel N, Staunton E, Goodchild L, Haslam RR, Dent J, et al. Paradoxical impact of body positioning on gastroesophageal reflux and gastric emptying in the premature neonate. J Pediatr. 2004;145:194–200.

153. Croft RD. What consistency of food is best for children with cerebral palsy who cannot chew? Arch Dis Child. 1992;67:269–71.

154. Cichero JAY, Nicholson TM, September C. Thickened mild for management of feeding and swallowing issues in infants: a call for interdisciplinary professional guidelines. J Hum Lact. 2012;29(2):132–5.

155. Scheel CE, Schanler RJ, Lau C. Does choice of bottle nipple affect the oral feeding performance of very-low-birthweight (VLBW) infants? Acta Paediatr. 2005;94:1266–72.

156. Taastrup R, Hansen BM, Kronborg H, Bojesen SN, Hallum K, Frandsen A, et al. Factors associated with exclusive breastfeeding of preterm infants. Results from a prospective national cohort study. PLOS One [Internet]. 2014;9(2):e89077.

157. Rogers B. Feeding method and health outcomes of children with cerebral palsy. J Pediatr. 2004;145(2 Suppl):S28–32.

158. Embleton ND. Early nutrition and later outcomes in preterm infants. In: Shamir R, Turck D, Philip M, editors. Nutrition and growth, World review of nutrition and diet, vol. 106. Basil: Karger; 2013.

159. Sleigh G, Brocklehurst P. Gastrostomy feeding in cerebral palsy: a systematic review. Arch Dis Child. 2004;89:534–9.

160. Dahlseng MO, Andersen GL, Andrada MDG, Arnaud C, Balu R, De La Cruz J, et al. Gastrostomy tube feeding of children with cerebral palsy: variation across six European countries. Dev Med Child Neurol. 2012;54(10):938–44.

161. Mason SJ, Harris G, Blissett J. Tube feeding in infancy: implications for the development of normal eating and drinking skills. Dysphagia. 2005;20:46–61.

162. Bazyk S. Factors associated with the transition to oral feeding in infants fed by nasogastric tubes. Am J Occup Ther. 1990;44(12):1070–8.

163. Fairhurst CBR, Cockerill H. Management of drooling in children. Arch Dis Child Educ Pract. 2011;96:25–30.

164. Scott A, Johnson HM. A practical approach to the management of saliva. 2nd ed. Austin: Pro-ed; 2004.

165. Cuvo AJ. Training children with autism and pervasive developmental disorders to comply with healthcare procedures: theory and research. In: Matson JL, Sturmey P, editors. International handbook of autism and pervasive developmental disorders. 2011. p. 381–95.

166. Arvedson JC, Clark H, Lazarus C, Schooling T, Frymark T. Evidence-based systematic review: effects of oral motor interventions on feeding and swallowing in preterm infants. Am J Speech Lang Pathol. 2010;19:321–40.

167. Fucile S, Gisel E, Lau C. Oral stimulation accelerates the transition from tube to oral feeding in preterm infants. J Pediatr. 2002;141(2):230–6.

168. Pinelli J, Symington A. Non-nutritive sucking for promoting physiologic stability and nutrition in preterm infants. Cochrane Database Syst Rev. 2005;19(4):CD001071.

169. Barlow SM, Finan DS, Lee J, Chu S. Synthetic orocutaneous stimulation entrains preterm infants with feeding difficulties to suck. J Perinatol. 2008;28:541–8.

170. Law-Morstatt L, Judd DM, Snyder P, Baier RJ, Dhanireddy R. Pacing as a treatment technique for transitional sucking patterns. J Perinatol. 2003;23:483–8.

171. Brown J, Kim C, Lim A, Brown S, Desai H, Volker L, et al. Successful gastrostomy tube weaning program using an intensive multidisciplinary team approach. J Pediatr Gastroenterol Nutr. 2014;58(6):743–9.

172. Sheppard JJ. Motor learning approaches for improving negative eating-related behaviors and swallowing and feeding skills in children. In: Preedy V, editor. International handbook of behavior, diet and nutrition. London: Springer; 2011.

173. Piazza CC. Feeding disorders and behavior: what have we learned? Dev Disabil Res Rev. 2008;14:174–81.

174. Gonzalez ML, Taylor T, Borrero CSW, Sangkavasi E. An individualized levels system to increase independent mealtime behavior in children with food refusal. Behav Intervent. 2013;28:143–7.
175. Pinnington L, Hegarty J. Effects of consistent food presentation on oral-motor skill acquisition in children with severe neurological involvement. Dysphagia. 2000;10:192–202.
176. Gisel E. Interventions and outcomes for children with dysphagia. Dev Disabil Res Rev. 2008;14:165–73.
177. Bailey RL, Angell ME. Effects of an oral-sensory/oral-motor stimulation/positive reinforcement program on the acceptance of nonpreferred foods by youth with physical and multiple disabilities. Phys Disabil Educ Related Serv. 2006;24(1):41–61.
178. Gisel E. Effect of oral sensorimotor treatment on measures of growth and efficiency of eating in the moderately eating-impaired child with cerebral palsy. Dysphagia. 1996;11:48–58.
179. Gisel E, Applegate-Ferrante T, Benson JE, Bosma JF. Effect of oral sensorimotor treatment on measures of growth, eating efficiency and aspiration in the dysphagic child with cerebral palsy. Dev Med Child Neurol. 1995;37:528–43.
180. Kim BR, Sung IY, Choi KH, Kim LS. Long-term outcomes in children with swallowing dysfunction. Dev Neurorehabil. 2014;17:298–305; Early online: 1–8.
181. Bandstra NF, Crist WB, Napier-Phillips A, Flowerdew G. The impact of behavioral feeding intervention on health care utilization. Child Health Care. 2011;40:282–96.

Presbyphagia

10

Dália Nogueira

Introduction

The demographic changes caused by the baby boomers are expected to alter the profile of the world's population. The number of older people continues to rise, particularly in industrialized countries. By the year 2020, it is estimated that 16.4 % of the population will be over the age of 65 [1], and a significant proportion of those older people will have a swallowing impairment [2]. It has been estimated that 13% to 35% of older people who live independently report dysphagic symptoms, with the vast majority failing to seek treatment [3]. Aging does not consist of an accumulation of diseases and is not synonymous with dependency. It is a process in which the organism starts to become frail. The term "homeostenose" refers to the decline in function with the reduction of the reserve margins; it is a process that begins to manifest itself in the third decade of life though varying greatly from one person to the other. The physiological and morphological changes in the organs and tissues that lead to their atrophy as well as to a decreased efficiency of the whole body system have strong functional implications. Furthermore, the organism is required to respond appropriately by adapting the physiologic and anatomic modifications to daily living requirements. The swallowing process is affected by these changes, and it is important to establish the frontiers between the normal and abnormal.

D. Nogueira, PhD, MSc, SLP
Speech and Language Therapy Department,
Escola Superior de Saúde de Alcoitão (ESSA) and Lisbon University Institute,
Praceta de Santa Cruz, 45, 2750-065 Areia, Cascais, Portugal
e-mail: dmsnogueira@gmail.com

© Springer India 2015
G. Mankekar (ed.), *Swallowing – Physiology, Disorders, Diagnosis and Therapy*,
DOI 10.1007/978-81-322-2419-8_10

Normal Swallowing in the Healthy Young Adult

Before establishing the limits between the normal and the abnormal, the change from young healthy swallowing to aging swallowing and to disturbed swallowing must first be described and understood.

The process of swallowing requires the conjugation of a complex series of psychological, sensory, and motor behaviors that are both voluntary and involuntary. The upper aerodigestive tract has two primary functions: breathing and swallowing. To safely execute swallowing, the upper aerodigestive tract must reconfigure a system that concentrates valves and moves air for the purposes of breathing and talking, into one that ceases airflow, and protects the airway while food, fluid, secretions, and medications are moved to ensure adequate nutrition and hydration. Normally, this complex process requires precise timing, supratentorial input, elicitation of five cranial nerves (V, VII, IX, X, and XII), and the critical cessation of breathing until pressures are generated and material is cleared into the upper tract [4]. Adult swallowing physiology is typically described as having three phases, even though swallowing is a dynamic and overlapping process. More recent literature [5] indicates the existence of five distinct stages (the anticipatory phase, the extraoral preparatory phase, the preparatory phase, the oral phase, and the esophageal phase). Generally, it helps to think of swallowing in terms of an oropharyngeal and an esophageal phase. The oropharyngeal phase can be divided into an oral stage, which is under voluntary control with cranial nerves V, VII, X, and XII, and a pharyngeal stage, which is largely involuntary with cranial nerves IX, X, and XII.

The oral stage begins with the preparatory phase where food or liquid is taken into the oral cavity, and salivation occurs to help its segregation. Food is initially taken into the mouth, and the labial seal allows the stripping of the bolus from a utensil; it contains the bolus in the oral cavity preventing leakage of intake. Food is lubricated through mixing with saliva and masticated into manageable, swallow-sized portions using a rotary lateral jaw motion and tongue manipulation until a cohesive bolus is formed. The intrinsic musculature of the tongue, innervated by the nerve XII, also helps to manipulate the bolus and facilitate mastication through a lateral rolling motion that elevates and presses the bolus against the hard palate.

Buccal tension and grooving of the tongue contain the bolus and prevent pooling in the lateral sulcus. The swallow-sized portion of food or liquid is then pushed to the posterior pharynx, which triggers the pharyngeal phase of deglutition in which more than 40 pairs of muscles and five cranial nerves are activated in rapid succession. The soft palate is first elevated to close off the nasopharynx preventing regurgitation and creating intraoral pressure. The larynx is pulled up and forward by the actions of the suprahyoid muscles. After this action, the soft palate swells forward, maintaining the bolus in range of the tongue's tip and opening the nasopharynx for breath. Anterior bulging of the soft palate prevents premature spillage into the pharynx. This last action signals receptors in the anterior tonsillar pillars, soft palate, and oropharynx to initiate the reflexive pharyngeal phase and clears food or liquid from the oral cavity. The triggering of the swallow reflex begins the pharyngeal stage so there is no interruption in bolus movement.

The pharyngeal phase has six critical components: (1) elevation and retraction of the soft palate for complete velopharyngeal closure, (2) superior and anterior movement of the hyoid bone and larynx, (3) laryngeal closure and cessation of breathing, (4) opening of the cricopharyngeal sphincter, (5) ramping of the tongue base, and (6) contraction from the top bottom of the pharyngeal constrictors.

During the pharyngeal phase, laryngeal closure occurs to ensure optimal airway protection. This event begins at the level of the true vocal folds and advances to the level of the false vocal folds, aryepiglottic folds, and epiglottis. When vocal fold closure occurs, the arytenoid cartilages tilt anteriorly, and the tongue base moves posteriorly to close the laryngeal vestibule. Vocal fold closure prevents aspiration or the entry of food or liquid into the trachea, below the level of the true vocal folds. Simultaneously, the intrinsic laryngeal muscles contract, and the epiglottis flips down to further protect the airway from the path of the oncoming bolus. The movement of the epiglottis occurs due to bolus pressure, muscular forces pressing downward, and the aforementioned pressure of the tongue base moving posteriorly and the elevation of the larynx. Along with the peristaltic muscular wave, pharyngeal peristalsis requires movements of the tongue and larynx to generate pressure within the pharynx during the swallowing process. Retraction of the tongue and lowering of the larynx at the end of the swallow increases pressure in the hypopharynx. The bolus is then overwhelmed and conducted by sequential contractions of the pharyngeal musculature, i.e., it is propelled through the upper esophageal sphincter (UES) by the pulling forces of the larynx.

Anatomically, the UES incorporates the cricopharyngeus (CP) muscle, as well as some of the lower fibers of the pharyngeal constrictor and of the esophagus. Inhibitory stimulation allows relaxation of the CP and opening of the sphincter during maximal anterior-superior hyoid elevation. The degree of relaxation depends on the size of the bolus. For the bolus to reach the esophagus successfully, the UES must open briefly to let it pass. This requires both relaxation of the cricopharyngeus and contraction of the suprahyoid muscles [6].

The esophagus is a muscular tube that begins at the cricoid cartilage and terminates in the stomach. After the UES has relaxed enough to allow bolus passage, it then closes to seal off and prevent the return of the fluid or food into the pharyngeal area. In the esophagus, peristalsis propels the food to the stomach. At the posterior of the esophagus, the lower esophageal sphincter (LES) opens and the contents of the esophagus are released. Once the bolus has passed, the UES closes and the esophageal circular muscle contracts sequentially. This in turn pushes the bolus toward the stomach. The LES then retroactively closes to prevent the return of the bolus into the esophagus, or gastroesophageal reflux, from occurring. Entry into the stomach is afforded by relaxation of the LES, which begins almost immediately after the initiation of swallowing and persists until the bolus has passed [7]. The vagus nerve mediates inhibition of this lower esophageal sphincter (LES) in response to bolus stimulation, as well as gastric distention. Passage of the bolus through the LES completes the act of deglutition. Although the coordination of most of the muscles involved in swallowing comes from the brainstem, the cerebral cortex is essential to the voluntary preparatory phase of swallow and portions of the pharyngeal phase. Input from both cerebral hemispheres maintains facial tone and prevents spillage from the mouth. Patterned movements, modulated by the cerebral cortex, govern bolus control and mastication during the preparatory phase. The brainstem houses the motor nuclei of most of all the muscles involved in swallowing, as well as the pattern generators necessary to trigger a complete swallowing reflex. The two brainstem regions most related to swallowing are the nucleus tractus solitarius and the nucleus ambiguus. The tractus solitarius receives both cortical and subcortical input, as well as peripheral sensory input through free nerve endings of glossopharyngeal and vagal afferent fibers within the oropharynx. Stimulus unleashed from these sources results in a coordinated swallow. The nucleus ambiguus houses the vagal motor nuclei and is responsible for the esophageal phase of swallowing. Although the trigger for primary peristalsis is the vagal nucleus, the intrinsic nerves of the esophagus propagate secondary, or autonomous, peristalsis from the junction between striated and smooth muscle fibers. Thus, central control of swallowing is maintained from the oral cavity to the midportion of the esophagus [6].

Physiology of Swallowing in Older People

The work focused on the anatomy and physiology of the oral and pharyngeal swallowing mechanism indicates a progression of change with age, which is combined with naturally diminished functional reserves. The ability to adapt to physiological stress makes older people more susceptible to dysphagia. Significant changes caused by the physiological aging process cause modifications in the organs and systems of swallowing, altering its normal performance. However, an older adult's swallow is not necessarily impaired. Presbyphagia refers to characteristic changes in the swallowing mechanism when comparing with those of healthy older adults. Older adults are more vulnerable and have an increased threat of acute illnesses, medication consumption, and any number of age-related conditions which can push them across the line from having a healthy older swallow to being dysphagic [8].

As people age, the swallowing mechanism shows significant differences, and the bolus transit may be disrupted, entering the lower airways (penetration or aspiration) or stopping [3]. Age-related alterations in swallowing have been extensively studied indicating minor changes in swallow function with normal aging. However, it is difficult to separate age-related phenomena from the effects of a disease. Atrophy and fibrosis of muscles that occur with aging result in a reduced range, speed, and accuracy of structural movement. Fat content in the tongue increases approximately 2.7 % per decade, possibly contributing to sarcopenia in the tongue. Laryngeal age-related changes are also noteworthy. The reduced motor unit firing rate, atrophy, and loss of laryngeal muscle fibers; ossification of laryngeal cartilage; increased irregularity of laryngeal cartilage auricular surfaces; and reduced sensation in the pharynx and larynx have all been documented as well as other characteristics related to the process of aging.

Oral Health Status

Older adults seem inclined to problems related to their oral health; the most common oral problems among older people are the loss of natural teeth, impaired ability to perform oral hygiene, loss of alveolar bone to support removable prostheses, and periodontal disease. There is a relationship between oral health and the risk of malnutrition in older people. These factors increase the probability of the co-occurrence of presbyglutition placing older people at even greater risk of dysphagia and malnutrition.

Dentition and Loss of Alveolar Bone

If dentition is good, the masticatory function remains good but with some increased chewing force necessary for bolus preparation. The continuum of dentition seen in older adults may range from retention of a full complement of teeth to full upper and lower dentures. Between these extremes are those with prosthetic or missing teeth. In a comparison of liquid swallows in edentulous and dentulous older adults, Yoshikava et al. [9] found that edentulous older people exhibited greater incidence of laryngeal penetration than dentate older people. The individuals with many missing teeth limit food choices due to chewing problems. Also, dentures will lack adherence to the mucosa and move around. Those with their own dentition and if dental caries are untreated, the bacteria associated with dental caries place someone who aspirates at greater risk of developing aspiration pneumonia.

Xerostomia dental issues and taste are the most common phenomena studied in relation to swallowing and eating status in older adults. Xerostomia actually has far reaching effects that can be seen in both dentition status and altered taste. By avoiding foods that require chewing, less saliva is produced, promoting a vicious circle between a downgrade of texture and the presence of xerostomia. Both dentulous and edentulous issues relate directly to xerostomia. Xerostomia can also promote dental caries because the immune functions of saliva are diminished, and the protective function of flora and fauna is disrupted.

Tongue

The tongue is the primary propulsive agent for pumping food through the mouth, into the pharynx while bypassing the airway, and through the esophagus. More substantial changes occur in the tongue because the lingual pressure reserve necessary to drive pharyngeal swallowing is diminished in older people. In addition, increased connective tissue within the body of the tongue restricts bolus control, requiring multiple tongue movements that hold the bolus more posteriorly and allow the bolus to enter the vallecula prematurely. Isometric tongue pressure in older adults is significantly less than that of younger subjects. The difference between isometric pressures is termed reserved pressure. Recent findings clearly reveal that an age-related change in lingual pressures is another contributing factor to presbyphagia. Although older individuals manage to achieve the pressure necessary to affect a successful swallow, despite a reduction in overall maximum tongue strength, it takes them longer than young swallowers. It has been suggested that the slowness that characterizes senescent swallowing may reflect the increased time necessary to recruit sufficient motor units to generate pressures necessary to operate an effective, safe swallow. The study of Youmans [10] showed that tongue strength reserve is lower in women than in men.

Masticatory Performance

The decrease of masticatory performance affects nutrient intake particularly in older people. Mastication is controlled by suprabulbar structures and consists of coordinated movements of masticatory organs such as the tongue, lips, cheeks, and mandible. Motor functions of these organs are known to deteriorate with age and to influence masticatory performance. However, there are only a few reports on the relationships between changes in tongue and lip function and masticatory performance with age [11]. Therefore, masticatory disorders might occur frequently as a result of oral motor dysfunction in older people.

Salivation

Mucus and saliva serve as positive and protective physiological purposes throughout the body. Mucosal tissues secrete mucus which acts like a moving blanket. Together, the mucosal tissue and its mucus covering create a layer of protection with the non-sterile external environment of the body. Mucus is an important component of saliva. The paired parotid, sublingual, and submaxillary glands as well as minor glands throughout the oral cavity produce saliva. Salivation can be stimulated as when eating or unstimulated as in a rest state. The act of mastication is a known stimulant of saliva production. The constituents vary in the two states. The functions of saliva are to begin the digestive process of carbohydrates; to maintain a moist mouth to aid chewing, swallowing, and speaking; and to act as an important participant in the immune system. As saliva mixes with food during chewing, it facilitates creation of homogeneous and malleable bolus and the retention of drier foods within that bolus. Oral transport of the bolus through the oral cavity and pharynx is facilitated by a wet bolus. Chronic dry mouth can be subjective (xerostomia) as well as objective (hyposalivation). Xerostomia, which often extends from the mouth to the pharynx and esophagus, can hinder bolus flow and result in the retention of material along the swallowing tract. Functional salivary production has been shown to remain stable throughout the age spectrum; however, older adults demonstrate decreased salivary reserve due to a loss of saliva production. Xerostomia increases with age and is experienced by approximately 30 % of the persons aged 65 years and older. Many authors believe that side effects of medication are the primary reason for xerostomia in older adults; this will be addressed later in the chapter. It is well known that certain classes of drugs promote dry mouth.

Taste

Taste appears to be essentially unchanged in aging, despite evidence of a change in taste buds and their related structures. Nevertheless, some older adults do complain that food does not taste the same. Possible causes of this taste dissatisfaction are full upper dental plates covering the hard palate, impaired chewing, and altered threshold for sour taste. Medication can add a metallic taste or diminish taste. Adding saliva to solids and fluids is necessary to maintain health and function of taste receptors. Xerostomia is thus another factor that contributes to taste change with age. In addition, saliva is the means by which taste substances are dissolved and then diffused to various taste receptor sites.

Weak Oral Movement

Structurally, sarcopenia is associated with age-related reductions in muscle mass and the cross-sectional area, a reduction in the number or size of muscle fibers, and a transformation or selective loss of specific muscle fiber types. Sarcopenia is inherently associated with diminished strength. The literature reports sarcopenia-like changes in muscles of the upper aerodigestive tract, and the observed age-related changes in strength and function suggest pervasive changes also in lingual muscle composition [4].

Reduced skeletal muscle strength is common in older people and leads to difficulty in cup drinking and mastication. There may be difficulty in ingesting, controlling, and delivering the bolus, as well as a significantly altered mastication impact in the oral phase; however, modified diet consistency and feeding duration often compensate oral phase impairment, which therefore lies, in most of the cases, silent. The pharyngeal phase is of greater clinical significance because of the risk of presenting aspiration phenomena; in order to avoid this risk, the young adult swallowing has an excess of strength and coordination, called swallowing reserve, which is significantly reduced in the older people. In fact, aging delays pharyngeal swallowing, and multiple swallows are required to clear a bolus from the pharynx in healthy older people. The probability of laryngeal penetration is also increased, because older people tend to inspire rather than expire after swallowing. Moreover, the reduced pharyngolaryngeal sensibility with age means that silent aspiration may occur as a consequence of reduced pharyngeal reserve. The esophageal phase also shows significant modifications; the secondary esophageal peristalsis, which cleans the esophageal residue after primary peristalsis, is in most cases absent.

Sensory Changes

Sensory input for taste, temperature, and tactile sensation changes in many older adults, e.g., sensory discrimination thresholds in the oral cavity and laryngopharynx have been shown to increase with age. This disruption of sensory-cortical-motor feedback ties may interfere with bolus formation and the timely response of the sensory-motor sequence, as well as detract from the pleasure of eating. Thus, reduced sensation may explain the failure of some older adults, such as those with dementia or Parkinson's disease, to spontaneously swallow when there is a pool of food, liquid, or saliva in the pharynx.

Pharyngeal Abnormalities

Pharyngeal phase abnormalities are of greater clinical significance because they reduce the swallowing reserve (a strength and coordination in excess of that needed to prevent aspiration). Despite the preservation of muscular activity, pharyngeal swallowing is more delayed in healthy older people than younger subjects, and older people frequently require multiple swallows to effectively clear a bolus from the pharynx. During this time, these subjects are three times more likely to inspire rather than expire after swallowing and have more laryngeal penetration as evidenced by coughing and multiphasic laryngeal movements. Coupled with the deficits in pharyngolaryngeal sensory discrimination that occur with age, this reduction in pharyngeal reserve may lead to silent aspiration. In older adults, the trigger of the pharyngeal swallow begins with the bolus in the valleculae for masticated materials and passes the ramus of the mandible for sequential liquid swallows. In young adults, however, initiation of the pharyngeal swallow begins at the anterior faucial pillars.

Esophageal Motility

Although some studies suggest that esophageal motor function deteriorates with age, other studies using more sophisticated recording techniques demonstrate minimal or no age-related changes in esophageal motility. The term presbyesophagus could be a misnomer and simply represent diffuse esophageal spasms in older people. Nevertheless, some researchers speculate that these changes result in decreased functional reserve, and therefore, problems develop more easily when disease or generalized weakness as a result of systemic illness intervenes [7]. Logemann [12] documented reduced neuromuscular reserve in older men and reduced flexibility in the cricopharyngeal opening as part of the normal aging of the motor system. Esophageal function shows moderate deterioration with slower transit and clearance. Equally threatening is the risk of residue within the esophagus traveling retrograde or refluxing from the esophagus into the pharynx and potentially the trachea.

Upper Esophageal Sphincter Function

Careful studies of the oropharyngeal phase of deglutition have identified impaired pharyngeal peristalsis and UES opening. Despite somewhat contradictory studies regarding normal changes in UES function as we age, decreased pharyngeal clearance may also be the result of CP and proximal esophageal abnormalities. Delayed exit of material from the pharynx may still occur, despite normal CP tone as a result of increased connective tissue in the UES and a decreased cross-sectional area of the esophageal accession. The abnormalities in the pharyngoesophageal transport may lead to longer feeding times, increased pharyngeal residue, and aspiration in some older patients [6].

Doty and Bosma [13] were among the first to note swallowing changes in older people. Despite numerous studies demonstrating physiological changes in swallowing with advancing age, there remains strong disagreement on what constitutes normal swallowing in older people and whether these changes represent dysphagia. Recent studies have indicated a number of discrete physiological changes in normal deglutition as we age. Overall, few clinically significant abnormalities arise during the oral phase, and feeding performance does not significantly worsen with age. As referred previously, most difficulties are caused by generalized age-related changes in skeletal muscle strength causing poor cup drinking and decreased masticatory strength. Although swallowing performance does not seem to be significantly affected by changes in oromotor skills, oral phase problems are common because difficulty ingesting, controlling, or delivering the bolus is noted in healthy older people. These abnormalities frequently remain silent because the individual effectively compensates by changing diet consistency and feeding duration. The longer swallow duration occurs largely before the more automatic pharyngeal swallow phase is initiated. Although the specific neural underpinning is not confirmed, it might be hypothesized that the more voluntary oral events become uncoordinated from the more "neural hard-wired" brainstem pharyngeal response which includes airway protection. Thus, it is not uncommon in older healthy adults for the bolus to be adjacent to an open airway for longer than in younger adults due to pooling or pocketing in the pharyngeal recesses, thus increasing the risk of adverse consequences caused by ineffective deglutition more frequent in old age [4].

In summary, the first signs of aging changes may begin as early as 45 years, namely, the age-associated alterations in the anatomical and physiological underpinnings of deglutition, biologically present but asymptomatic, thus entering a preclinical state. Initially, these changes in swallowing are unlikely to interfere with functional nutrition or hydration. However, there is a point in the deterioration where cumulative changes of presbyphagia transition to dysphagia, even without a specific medical condition. The emergence of the clinical state is reached when dysphagia is symptomatic and detectable through routine care.

It is increasingly critical that health professionals are able to distinguish between dysphagia and presbyphagia in order to avoid overdiagnosing and overtreating dysphagia. Older adults can be more vulnerable to dysphagia, primarily with additional stressors such as acute illnesses and certain medications. The presence of such stressors can result in a healthy older swallow (presbyphagia) crossing over the line to experiencing dysphagia. It is essential for healthcare professionals to be alert in order to correctly diagnose dysphagia and treat it in a timely manner [4].

Changes in Normal Swallow with Age
- Changes as the resulting forms of illness and subsequent general weakness
- Cricopharyngeal opening diameter across volumes reduced
- General weakness

- Hyoid and laryngeal maximum vertical movement significantly reduced
- Hyoid and laryngeal movements slower up to the time of cricopharyngeal opening virtually
- Increased frequency of inspiration (instead of expiration) after swallowing
- Increased oral and pharyngeal residue
- Increased swallowing apnea duration
- Muscles with reduced strength
- Penetration and aspiration occurs more frequently
- Pharyngeal delay times (contraction inconsistently slower)
- Pharyngeal phase delayed, i.e., trigger of the swallowing reflex
- Reduced fall in the number of deglutitions per minute
- Reduced flexibility
- Reduced laryngeal elevation and sensibility
- Reduced number of teeth
- Reduced opening of the upper esophageal sphincter
- Reduced oral sensibility
- Reduced oral stereognostic abilities
- Reduced pharyngeal peristalsis width and velocity
- Reduced reserve – especially in men
- Reduced tongue pressure and coordination of lingual muscles
- Residue is generally only slightly greater
- Safety of swallow normally unchanged
- Timing of the swallow: oral transit times slightly but significantly longer in older adults

Dysphagia in Older People

Plurimorbidity and dysphagia are commonly found to be a major problem in older people. In particular, diseases causing dysphagia, diet and functional modifications induced by aging, and the use of medications often coexist in the same individual. Some previous studies have reported a significant decline in swallowing function among frail or impaired older people [12, 14]. These results suggest that it is necessary to determine the risk of dysphagia for frail older people in community dwellings. Several researchers have demonstrated that the following variables are effective predictors of dysphagia and aspiration: delayed oral transit, incomplete oral clearance, change of voice quality, abnormal gag reflex, and abnormal voluntary cough [15]. When dysphagia is due not only to the aging mechanism but also to a pathological mechanism, the term secondary presbyphagia is used. At best, changes in swallowing function can affect enjoyment and social interactions. At worst, complications can include dehydration, malnutrition, weight loss, and aspiration pneumonia and may significantly impact the length of stay and cost of care for both acute and long-term patients. Risk factors affecting the ability to swallow for the geriatric population are varied considering the mechanical, neurologic, and mental status changes common in this age group.

In recent years, much has been written on the etiologies and the physiologic mechanisms of dysphagia, as well as on the advances in diagnostic and therapeutic options for the disorder. However, there is little or no information on dysphagia in older persons who have no comorbidities. Presbyglutition will deteriorate to dysphagia in some older people but not others. Although the older person with comorbidities is more likely to develop swallowing problems, the ambiguity of when and in whom dysphagia will manifest itself makes it difficult to anticipate and to recognize the problem. In general, dysphagia in the older population is no different from dysphagia in any other subject. However, older patients sometimes do not communicate their symptoms adequately and are more likely than younger patients to present with recurrent aspiration pneumonia without being aware of dysphagia [7].

Signs and symptoms related to swallowing disorders are listed above. If a person with dysphagia aspirates, he or she is at risk of developing aspiration pneumonia, especially when other factors such as acid reflux and dental caries are present. Aspiration pneumonia is one of the factors associated with treatment failure in patients with community-acquired pneumonia. Those with dysphagia often have great difficulty drinking thin liquids, and water can pose the greatest problem because of its characteristic neutral taste and lack of texture. Thus, individuals with dysphagia are more likely to be dehydrated. Dehydration can have numerous consequences such as constipation, falls, and respiratory infections and is associated with morbidity and mortality in older adults. If dysphagia is added to such a scenario, then dehydration is even more likely.

Some of the major alterations related to swallowing disorders:

- Alteration of voice quality during or after eating
- Aspiration with reduced sensitivity
- Avoidance of certain foods because of swallowing problems
- Avoidance of eating in company
- Reflux esophageal-pharyngeal seconds after swallowing
- Changes in approach to food
- Choking, coughing before, during, or after eating
- Compensatory measures intuitively adopted (head and neck movements)
- Complaints of food in the throat after posterior glottic erythema or edema
- Complaints of food/liquid going the wrong way due to incomplete glottal closure
- Aspiration with good sensitivity
- Spillage before swallowing
- Cough immediately (including generalized weakness)
- Residue in vestibule aspirated on inhalation after swallowing
- Complains that food sticks in the throat
- Coughing when lying down or after meals
- Coughing, throat clearing, or choking before, during, or after eating
- Difficulty initiating a swallow
- Difficulty placing food in the mouth
- Difficulty swallowing liquids

- Difficulty swallowing medication
- Difficulty swallowing solids
- Drooling or oral spillage; pooling and pocketing of food
- Dry mouth
- Dysarthria
- Dysfunction of focal musculature
- Esophageal or gastric reflux
- Fasciculations
- Food "sticking" in the throat or chest
- Food coming out of nose during eating (regurgitation) due to velopharyngeal incompetence
- Food spillage from the mouth
- Forcibly regurgitating food that is stuck in the throat
- Frequent throat clearing
- Gurgly or wet voice
- Hoarse, breathy voice; incomplete glottal closure and penetrations, aspiration before or during the swallow
- Ineffective cough/clearing
- Hypernasal voice: velopharyngeal (v/ph) closure deficit, nasal reflux
- Impaired breathing during meals or immediately after eating
- Inability to control food, liquid, or saliva in the mouth
- Inability to handle secretions
- Increase amount of food remaining on plate
- Increased mucous or phlegm in the throat before, during, or after eating
- Increased need to clear throat
- Intermittent cessation of intake, frequent "wash downs"
- Laborious chewing, repetitive swallowing
- Lack of awareness or reaction: no spontaneous clearing or reduced awareness or reaction to spillage, penetration to wet voice secretions; impaired sensitivity when probed aspiration of residue
- Leakage of food or saliva from tracheostomy site
- Takes a long time to eat because of swallowing problem
- Manifestations of impaired oropharyngeal functions
- Neck pain, chest pain, or heartburn
- Need to chew excessively in order to swallow safely
- No complaint but coughs severally: reduced sensation to touch of endoscope
- Pain on swallowing
- Pain or pressure in the throat or chest during swallowing
- Rapid respiratory rate: cannot sustain glottal closure more than a few seconds; no airway protection during spillage; aspiration before, during, or after swallowing, especially with fatigue
- Recurrent pneumonia or exacerbation of asthma
- Regurgitation of food or acid
- Regurgitation of food or pills
- Residual food in the oral cavity

- Sensation of food sticking in the throat
- Sensation of obstruction of the bolus in throat or chest
- Sense of difficulty initiating the swallow
- Sneezing during or after meal
- Special physical preparation of food or avoidance of foods of specific consistency
- Taking smaller bites of food in order to swallow safely
- Throat clearing
- Unexplained weight loss
- Weak cough: incomplete glottal closure; poor sustained aspiration during swallow; ineffective clearance; breath holding if aspirates
- Wet voice quality: secretions/food residue in retrocrichoid region; penetration/aspiration of liquid food
- Wet, hoarse voice, and other voice changes
- Gasping after eating

Few studies examine dysphagia or oral problems as potential risk factors in malnutrition in community-dwelling older people. Compromised nutrition from poor eating can decrease resistance to infection, exacerbate disease, result in longer hospital stays, and increase complications and disability. In fact, nutritional risk factors such as a 5 % or greater weight loss in community-dwelling older adults are an important predictor of institutionalization.

As such, major adjustments in the process of swallowing, eating, and drinking can lead to distressing responses such as shame, anxiety, depression, and isolation. Dysphagia profoundly influences quality of life (QOL) [4].

Several disorders with a higher incidence in the geriatric population can cause dysphagia, putting older people at greater risk of aspiration. Side effects of many commonly used medications can also contribute to dysphagia and as previously referred cause dry mouth, tardive dyskinesia, drowsiness, or suppressed gag or cough reflex [16].

Dysphagia in older people is often found in conjunction with neurologic conditions, such as stroke, Parkinson's disease, Alzheimer's dementia, and other dementia syndromes, and head and neck tumors or cancer. Patients with esophageal dysphagia complain of pain in the chest area after swallowing. Common causes of esophageal dysphagia include esophagitis, strictures, achalasia (ineffective relaxation of the LES), and esophageal spasm. Dysfunction may occur during any phase of the swallowing process, causing dysphagia. Effective cranial nerve function is paramount to optimal swallowing, and less obvious yet still prevalent conditions such as poor dentition, gastroesophageal reflux disorder (GERD), and even the common cold can result in weight loss and swallowing problems.

Neurologic diseases rise in prevalence in older population cohorts with its consequences: between 50 and 75 % of patients who have had a recent acute stroke develop eating and swallowing problems, and ensuing complications of aspiration develop in 50 %, malnutrition in 45 %, and pneumonia in 35 %. Brainstem or bilateral hemispheric strokes predictably produce dysphagia, but unilateral lesions also can contribute to this. A host of common problems involving the head and neck can directly damage the effector muscles of swallowing and increase the risk of dysphagia. Head and neck injury, carcinoma, complex infections, thyroid conditions, and diabetes are associated with age-related dysphagia. Although vertebral osteophytes are common, they rarely cause dysphagia. Dysphagia more commonly results from the presence of osteophytes in conjunction with neuromuscular weakness or in coordination. This can be caused by combinations of several underlying conditions or comorbidities such as diabetes, chronic obstructive pulmonary disease, congestive heart failure, renal failure, an immunocompromised status, and/or cachexia so that for which an individual can no longer draw an adequate reserve to effectively compensate. Sometimes, dysphagia can have iatrogenic causes. Healthcare interventions can result in drug-induced delirium, protracted hospital stays, and ultimately malnutrition. Indwelling nasogastric tubes, airway intubation, and medication effects may all predispose a frail older adult with borderline airway protection to developing frank aspiration. Understanding the iatrogenic causes of dysphagia can alter medical practice and may reduce its incidence and complications [4].

One of the most common age diseases is Parkinson disease (PD) that is characterized by loss of striatal dopamine, and hand tremors can make self-feeding difficult or impossible. As the disease progresses, cranial nerve function may be affected, causing speech and swallowing difficulties. Delays in the oral preparatory, oral transport, and esophageal phases are found in most patients; other dysphagia findings include reduced laryngeal elevation, complete glottal closure, delayed triggering of pharyngeal swallowing and UES relaxation. This results in pooling in the valleculae and pyriform sinuses. Reduced laryngeal elevation and movement of the base of the tongue can cause dysfunction at the cricopharyngeal juncture or upper esophageal sphincter. This creates a risk of aspiration after the completion of the swallow. Repetitive movements and rigidity typical in Parkinson's can affect the oral stage resulting in difficulty moving the bolus.

Dementia

When discussing the phases of swallowing, the division of oral, pharyngeal, and esophageal is the typically described. However, some other (sub) phases are also important. The anticipatory stage recognizes cognitive, affective, motor, and sensory stimuli that precede the oral preparatory stage of swallowing. Although first described more than a decade ago, this stage of swallowing is discussed less frequently in the swallowing literature. Specific examples include sensory stimulus such as smell and appearance of food as well as premeal rituals. It also includes the hand-to-mouth aspects of eating and the modification of oral postures to accept various utensils. It is asserted that the anticipatory stage is a necessary precursor to the execution of physiological swallowing. Without it, sequential aspects of swallowing will not transpire smoothly. The anticipatory stage of swallowing is particularly vulnerable in patients with cognitive deficits. These problems will vary with the type as well as the progress of dementia. Impaired memory may result in forgotten meals, and distractions in the environment can interfere with a patient's focus on the process of eating. Moreover, lack of recognition of food (agnosia) may result in a prolonged oral phase. All of these issues can dispose patients with dementia to malnutrition, dehydration, and aspiration. Thus, monitoring at mealtimes in this population is advocated [17].

Chronic Obstructive Pulmonary Disease

Chronic obstructive pulmonary disease (COPD) is an important risk factor. As respiration and swallowing are closely integrated and coordinated, it is possible that the changes in respiratory function that occur with COPD may produce swallowing problems. However, few studies have examined the nature of the swallowing problems in patients with COPD, and the frequency of swallowing disorders in this population is not well known. Difficulty with airway closure and aspiration during the swallow has been reported in COPD, as well as gastroesophageal reflux.

Cricopharyngeal Dysfunction

One of the more perplexing causes of dysphagia in older people is *cricopharyngeal* (CP) dysfunction. This difficulty begins with the discrepancy between the physiological sphincter and its muscular components. Functional CP disorders result from partial or complete failure of UES relaxation. Commonly seen in association with neurological disorders affecting the upper aerodigestive tract, functional UES disorders are characterized by a delayed or incomplete opening of the cricopharyngeal segment with bolus stasis at the level of the hypopharynx. Functional CP disorders may be seen following brainstem strokes (Wallenberg syndrome), after head trauma, or in association with neurodegenerative diseases. In contrast to the failed sphincter relaxation of functional CP disorders, Individuals with structural abnormalities of the UES demonstrate delayed or incomplete opening of the cricopharyngeal segment despite normal relaxation.

Medication

Older people frequently report difficulty swallowing pills as the first sign of a swallowing problem. Polypharmacy in old age is routine practice as the incidence of certain medical conditions become chronic and it increases with age. While difficulty swallowing pills can be an indicator of dysphagia, the drugs themselves can be part of the problem. A large number of medications, spanning several classes of pharmacological agents, have undesirable effects on swallowing. Drugs can cause xerostomia or influence LES relaxation and reflux via anticholinergic mechanisms. An equally large number affect cognition and mental status or influence the tongue and bulbar musculature by delaying neuromuscular responses or inducing extrapyramidal effects, which can hinder safe and sufficient oral intake [4]. Dryness of the mouth impairs bolus transport, resulting in increased residual in both the oral cavity and oropharynx. Saliva also contains bicarbonate that helps neutralize stomach acid and protect the esophagus and hypopharynx from chemical injury. Because saliva production is controlled by parasympathetic stimulation, xerostomia results from all medications with significant anticholinergic activity. The following common classes of drugs have anticholinergic side effects: antihistamines, tricyclic antidepressants, neuroleptics, antiemetics, atropine-containing antidiarrheal agents, and anti-parkinsonian medications. In addition to direct cholinergic interference on saliva production, diuretics frequently indirectly aggravate xerostomia through dehydration. Many medications that alter or depress central nervous system activity may cause dysphagia in older patients. Anxiolytics such as benzodiazepines, commonly used for sleep disorders, are often metabolized slowly in older patients and may be associated with dysphagia. Alcohol, found in many over-the-counter medication preparations, has an identical effect and predisposes to gastroesophageal reflux through LES relaxation [6, 18].

Environment and Swallowing Disorders in Older People

While well characterized in acutely ill populations, the prevalence and quality-of-life changes associated with dysphagia remain poorly defined in the community geriatric population. In older people, feeding can be affected not only by primary and secondary presbyphagia but also by the environment in which the person lives. As aging and diseases impair swallowing, other systems should be employed to ensure appropriate feeding: the physical environment should reduce interfering stimuli, appropriate food consistency should be provided, and, when hand-to-mouth movement is impaired, caregivers should feed the older people using adequate timing and bolus volume. In older people with dysphagia, additional cognitive resources to the automatic cerebral circuits need to be employed in order for the food to be swallowed properly. Visual and acoustic stimuli, such as television or being in a large dining room, may diminish the level of attention and concentration and interfere with the delicate swallowing mechanism the older people person would achieve in a quiet environment. In the vast majority of both primary and secondary presbyphagia cases, the strategy that allows safe swallowing is diet modification. In order to implement diet modifications in everyday life, the compliance of the patient and the people involved in cooking and serving the food is needed. Difficulties in reaching this goal are related to the personal tastes of the patient and the social role of mealtime in older people. In fact, older patients may not accept a change in diet because the food is not tasty or they refuse to have their meal separately from the family. Furthermore, the people cooking the meals, both at home and in institutions, need to be taught the food consistency required – usually by speech and language pathologists. Moreover, diet modifications often require complex cooking so that the food remains appealing; this is not always achievable, especially in long-term settings. A final, important consideration is reserved to people who cannot feed themselves independently; in this population, the caregiver should respect the patient's breathing pattern when feeding and give him or her the extra time required.

When these goals are not achieved, the older people with dysphagia are exposed to an increased risk of complications. For instance, it has been recently shown that clinical factors, e.g., cognitive impairment; sociocultural factors, e.g., inability to speak; and institutional factors, e.g., an inadequate number of knowledgeable staff, contribute to inadequate fluid intake [3].

Dysphagia can also reduce opportunities for socialization. Persons with dysphagia may be embarrassed to eat with friends or in restaurants because of coughing or choking, which may result in increased loneliness and isolation. Over 50 % of persons with known dysphagia reported that they ate less than before, and 44 % had experienced weight loss in the last 12 months. Although 84 % felt that eating should be pleasurable, only 45 % found that it was so. More than a third (36 %) indicated they avoided eating with others, and 41 % indicated that they experienced anxiety or panic during mealtimes [17].

Dysphagia Assessment

Despite a greater understanding of swallowing physiology and advances in dysphagia evaluation, disorders of swallowing and feeding remain underappreciated by both the general public and physicians. There is some nescience therapeutic toward the problem of dysphagia in older people, primarily because the underlying cause is often not specifically treatable. A multidisciplinary approach is necessary for effective diagnosis and treatment of dysphagia in older people whether they are living in a community or an extended care facility. This holistic approach to diagnosis and management should include the physician, speech therapist, dietitian, nursing staff and caregivers, dentist, pharmacist, occupational therapist, and social worker. While reviewing the history, physicians should note weight loss, aspiration pneumonia, recurrent urinary tract infection, and so forth. The examination should include testing of cranial nerves, an otolaryngology examination, blood work to detect early signs of malnutrition or dehydration, and a review of all drugs and their effect on the swallowing mechanism. Assessment of mobility should consider the patient's ability to shop, prepare meals, and self-feed. If dysphagia is suspected, the speech therapist should be consulted.

A number of diagnostic tests and screening methods have been developed to find and treat dysphagia at an early stage; these include the repetitive saliva-swallowing test (RSST) [19], the 3-oz water swallowing test [20], oximetry, videofluorography, and videoendoscopy. Many of these tests are difficult to conduct noninvasively in an epidemiological survey, since most were designed for use in hospital settings. A few inventories of screening methods for dysphagia among community-dwelling older people living at home have also been made. Dysphagia risk assessment for the community-dwelling older people scores was significantly related to 3-oz water test, suggesting that it is a valid assessment tool for evaluating the risks associated with swallowing disorders [15].

The difficulty in diagnosing dysphagia in older people is multifactorial. Depression, cognitive function, and behavioral changes may delay the recognition of dysphagia. In addition, swallowing disorders are often insidious in their onset and may not manifest clinically for years or decades. Over such time periods, self-learned compensatory strategies mask the normal physiological changes that weaken the integrity of deglutition as we age. Although these changes have previously been described as "presbyphagia" and considered a natural part of senescence, the ability to adapt gradually to changes in eating and swallowing makes the diagnosis of dysphagia abnormal at any age. As such, the identification of swallowing disorders in older patients requires a comprehensive evaluation to determine the cause or origin and direct therapy. Recent advances in the evaluation of dysphagia allow specific anatomical and physiological abnormalities during deglutition to be identified. Although this information is useful to demonstrate the site of dysfunction, the origin or cause of a patient's dysphagia may remain obscure without a basic understanding of the complex physiology of deglutition and the changes that occur with normal aging [6].

Dysphagia in older people is a common finding in everyday clinical practice; appropriate assessment is based on the knowledge of the swallowing physiology and pathology and adequate interpretation of noninstrumental and instrumental findings provided by FEES and VFS. Careful examination of the clinical picture together with environmental facilitators and barriers is recommended in order to prevent dysphagia complications. Dysphagia assessment in this population relies primarily on the same modalities as in other age groups: history, bedside examination, fibrotic endoscopic examination of swallowing (FEES), and videofluoroscopy (VFS).

FEES relies on flexible fiberoptic laryngopharyngoscopy to assess dynamic swallowing abnormalities and aspiration. By using liquids and solids of different consistencies combined with dye colors, elements of pharyngeal swallowing may be examined directly for pathological changes. In a normal swallow, the bolus may not even be seen in the pharynx prior to swallowing, and there is no residue of material after the swallow; because of lingual, velar, and pharyngeal tissue crush against the tip of the endoscope, a whiteout of the view occurs during the pharyngeal phase. The salient abnormal findings that are most common are spillage before the swallow, residue after the swallow, laryngeal penetration, and tracheal aspiration. Even if the information obtained through FEES is limited compared to that of VFS, FEES is becoming increasingly popular, particularly in Europe, because of the low cost and the possibility of examining patients in different settings, even at the bedside. VFS, considered the "gold standard" for swallowing assessment, provides a dynamic view of deglutition from the oral cavity to the LES. Compensatory swallowing strategies may also be assessed. During VFS, each swallowing phase can be properly studied; the most important abnormal findings that can be observed during VFS are drooling, prolonged oral preparation time, tongue pumping deficits, inefficiency of serial swallows, oral stasis, poor mastication, nasal regurgitation, tracheal aspiration, laryngeal penetration, delayed initiation of swallowing, reduced hyoid and/or laryngeal elevation, vallecular stasis, deviant epiglottic function, pyriform sinus stasis, reduced laryngeal closure, and the presence of a cricopharyngeal bar. Drawbacks of this technique include exposure to radiation, requirement of multiple personnel (radiologist, SLT), limited availability, and relatively high costs. Videotaping allows a frame-by-frame analysis of motility, residue, and aspiration. The SLT assists the radiologist during the study. The speech therapist's report describes any abnormality of structures or movement, adequacy of valving, aspiration, efficacy of treatment techniques, and ultimately the patient's candidacy for oral feeding. Recommendations for diet modification, feeding procedures, positioning, and use of adaptive feeding devices are also included. Videoendoscopy or fiberoptic endoscopic evaluation of swallowing is also used to evaluate structures and image the pharynx before and after a swallow. Closure of the pharyngeal walls around the lens eliminates the image during the swallow. A flexible scope is inserted through the nose after the application of a light topical anesthetic. The oral stage of swallow cannot be observed. However, a good image can be obtained of the velopharyngeal closure and the pharynx. Pooling of secretion or residue can be seen, and pharyngeal sensitivity can also be assessed by the flexible endoscopic evaluation of swallowing with sensory testing.

Older people not only have different diseases and live in different environments, but they often show differences in anatomy and physiology; specialists involved in swallowing assessment should take all of these into consideration. In fact, the management of older patients with dysphagia should rely on specific criteria that do not completely overlap with those used for the young or adult patient with dysphagia [3]. Relying on individuals' self-report may result in under-recognition of some symptoms and overestimation of others. For some individuals with dysphagia, additional testing is critical. However, for other patients, trouble swallowing does not seem to be a worry. In that case, a watchful approach may be the best. Patient concern and experience of frequency, duration, and life interference are critical variables in determining the treatment decisions, testing, and use of medications. With up to one fifth of the population experiencing frequent difficulty swallowing, primary care physicians should remain alert to the presence of dysphagia in their patients but may need to consider multiple approaches [21].

Evaluation of swallowing disorders in older patients begins with a comprehensive history and physical examination. The first important determination to be made is whether the patient has a feeding or a swallowing disorder or both. Although such a distinction may seem simple, in practice, it can be difficult to elucidate. Questions regarding eating habits, duration of feeding, diet, frequency of meals, and weight changes are essential. Careful attention is paid to the patient's description of his or her dysphagia, food consistencies that are problematic, and onset pattern. Patients commonly use phrases like "It gets stuck in my throat," or "I just can't get it down." They should be asked to indicate where they feel food "sticking," and they generally give an accurate indication of the site of pooling (valleculae, pyriform sinus, or upper esophagus). Patients are also asked about odynophagia (pain during swallowing) and appetite. Patients with feeding problems secondary to cognitive difficulties may eat sporadically for short periods. Meal times are often irregular, and many of these patients progressively lose weight. Individuals with primary dysphagia often require longer feeding periods as they gradually adapt through strategies such as multiple swallows, smaller bites, and prolonged chewing. Once the diagnosis of dysphagia is suspected, it is not uncommon for physicians to turn their attention to physical examination and testing. However, careful questioning focused on many of the common characteristics of dysphagia can lead to a diagnosis in many cases. The presence of solid, semisolid, or liquid dysphagia can help direct the discussion immediately, demonstrating that, in general, individuals with fixed obstructions complain of solid rather than liquid dysphagia. Episodic dysphagia for both liquids and solids from the outset suggests a motor disorder, whereas deteriorating dysphagia that occurs initially in response to solids, such as meat and bread, and then progresses to semisolids and liquids, suggests a structural cause. Associated symptoms including nasopharyngeal regurgitation and dysarthria may point to the level of the lesion. Breathy hoarseness may represent glottic incompetence, which places the patient at risk of aspiration in the setting of other neurological abnormalities (e.g., decreased sensation or poor cough). Although wet vocal quality is commonly thought to be a symptom of swallowing incompetence, there is controversy over its importance. Whereas dysphonia has been associated with aspiration following acute stroke, wet vocal quality alone failed to demonstrate significant association with aspiration on videofluoroscopy. Thus, voice changes may be useful during bedside examination to evaluate swallowing function and response to therapy, but it is insufficient to predict aspiration in the absence of more objective studies. Completion of the dysphagia history includes a comprehensive review of systems and discussion of current medications. This information may point to other comorbid conditions affecting appetite, feeding behavior, or swallowing. Physical examination of the oral cavity and upper aerodigestive tract in conjunction with neurological evaluation focusing on mental status and cranial nerves can be useful in diagnosis and management of patients with dysphagia. Assessment should begin with an evaluation of the oral cavity and integrity of the oral mucosa. The presence of dental plates should be noted because denture wearers demonstrate a significant decrease in feeding performance that is independent of age; reflexes; oral sensitivity; range of motion; strength; and precision of labial, lingual, and velar movements. Attention to vocal quality gives an indication of vocal cord function and the need for examination by an otolaryngologist. If the patient is considered a candidate for trial with oral feeding, small amounts of puree, solid, thick, and thin liquid consistencies are given. Observation during the oral stage provides information about containment, ability to form bolus, oral transit time, struggle behavior, oral clearance, or presence of residue after completion of swallow. The clinician positions fingers lightly at four points (behind mandible, thyroid bone, and above and below the thyroid cartilage) to assess movement during the swallow and give a rough estimate of the pharyngeal trigger. Throat clearing and coughing before, during, or after completion of swallow provide indirect evidence of aspiration and pooling. For instance, "wet" vocal quality after completion of swallow is a soft sign of aspiration or pooling at the level of the larynx. The amount of energy expended during the feeding process and signs of fatigue is also noted because they may affect the amount of intake during a meal.

Saliva quantity and quality should be assessed because moisture is essential, not only for bolus formation but also as a trigger of the pharyngeal swallow through glossopharyngeal afferents. Neurological evaluation should include an assessment of the patient's level of arousal, orientation, and cognitive skills and thorough cranial nerve examination. Swallowing competence depends on skeletal muscle and, as such, is subject to weakness with diminished arousal states. Cranial nerve evaluation should focus on trigeminal (V), facial (VII), glossopharyngeal (IX), vagus (X), and hypoglossal (XII) cranial nerve function. Facial (VII) or tongue (XII) weakness may cause oral preparatory delays and become evident through anterior loss of bolus, premature bolus leakage over the tongue base, and increased oral residual. Similar findings may be noted in patients with sensory loss within the oral cavity through trigeminal nerve weakness or progressive loss of two-point discrimination. Gag reflex testing is a common component of the cranial nerve examination and assesses both glossopharyngeal sensation in the posterior pharyngeal wall and soft palate and vagus nerve motor function with velar movement, glottic closure, and hyoid elevation. Although gag reflex testing provides information about numerous components of deglutition, the significance of a poor gag response with regard to swallowing competence is less clear. It is important to note that the gag reflex is not a part of normal deglutition and is absent in more than one third of healthy adults without dysphagia. Confounding problems, such as diminished laryngeal sensation and poor cough, render bedside swallowing evaluation inadequate to assess pharyngeal and esophageal dysphagia or predict aspiration. Numerous noninvasive procedures, including respiratory pattern monitoring, pulse oximetry, cough reflex, ultrasonography, and acoustic monitoring, have been developed to assist the physician and the speech therapist in identifying patients with swallowing incompetence [6].

As referred above, bedside swallowing evaluation has long been criticized for its lack of accuracy in identifying aspirating patients. However, the implementation of a straightforward bedside assessment highlights the importance of having a simple screening tool for dysphagia that can be easily applied by health professionals involved in the care of older patients. The degree of agreement between the doctor's diagnosis of dysphagia and the diagnosis made by the speech therapist suggests that a simple bedside swallowing assessment which includes the finding of cough on swallowing and delayed swallowing will be useful as a screening tool for swallowing dysfunction in the hospitalized older patient [17].

During these assessments, the patient is monitored for signs of coughing and choking and to determine whether one texture of solid or thickness of liquid is better tolerated than another.

As food and eating play important cultural and psychosocial roles in this society, not to mention vital nutritional functions, clinicians are encouraged to remain informed about the evaluation and treatment of geriatric dysphagia. Utilizing a dysphagia-specific instrument can enhance clinical assessment; a direct "review of system" question on swallowing difficulties may not be sufficiently sensitive to identify quality-of-life impairments. Finally, more education and awareness on age-related swallowing disorders are needed in the community [22].

Dysphagia Management (Table 10.1)

Traditionally, interventions for dysphagia in older patients are compensatory in nature and are directed at modifying bolus flow by targeting neuromuscularly induced pathobiomechanics or by adapting the environment.

The growing interest in underlying mechanisms of strength-training exercises for dysphagia is particularly applicable to older people because of documented sarcopenia in this population. Exercise can be of benefit by means of muscle strengthening leading to an enhanced swallowing function. It can be of benefit in persons who remain in the preclinical stage of presbyglutition by helping to reestablish reserve. Individuals can participate in therapy to strengthen pharyngeal and oral musculature to reduce the adverse effects of muscular and sensory impairment. Depending on the area(s) of weakness, oral and pharyngeal muscle-strengthening exercises will be performed.

A compendium of studies has demonstrated that exercise regimens can promote change in swallowing in robust older adults. Lingual-resistant exercise promoted increased isometric and swallowing pressure in a group of healthy older adults. A subgroup in this study also underwent pre- and postexercise magnetic resonance imaging, and an increase in lingual volume was noted in each participant. In a study of the effects of the Shaker exercise, about half of the older people demonstrated an increase in anterior and superior movement of the hyoid bone between the mandible and the larynx, facilitating laryngeal elevation and upper esophageal sphincter opening. It can be difficult to know when an individual might benefit from swallowing diagnostic techniques or intervention strategies. Although speech therapists typically rely on patients, the community-dwelling older people may be overlooked [23].

For older people, treatment may include a variety of compensatory and rehabilitative techniques. Positioning the patient can compensate for weak structures and increase airway protection.

Swallowing therapists believe compensatory strategies are less demanding on the patient in terms of effort. These strategies include postural adjustment, slowing the rate of eating, limiting bolus size, adaptive equipment, and the most commonly used environment adaptation, diet modification. Postural adjustments are relatively simple to teach to a patient, require little effort to employ, and can eliminate misdirection of bolus flow through biomechanical adjustment. A general postural rule for facilitating safe swallowing is to eat in an upright posture (90° seated) so that the vertical phases (pharyngeal) of the oropharyngeal swallow as well as esophageal motility capitalize on gravitational forces. Upright posture also can assist in precluding early spillage of food or liquid from the horizontal oral phase into the pharynx and a potentially open airway as well as diminishing the probability of nasal regurgitation. A less obvious postural adjustment is useful for patients with hemiparesis. For this group of patients, a common strategy is a head turn toward the hemiparetic side, effectively closing that side off to bolus entry and facilitating bolus transit through the non-paretic pharyngeal channel. If the pathophysiologic condition is the uncoupling of the oral from the pharyngeal phase of the swallow

Table 10.1 Techniques used in dysphagia management and their expected results

Problem	Technique	Result
Residues in the pyriform sinus and alteration in pressure	Head rotated	Pulls cricoid cartilage away from posterior pharyngeal wall, reducing residue in pyriform sinuses and resting pressure
Bolus entering the airway	Chin down	Widens valleculae to prevent bolus entering airway; narrows airway entrance; pushes epiglottis posteriorly
Poor sensitivity in the pharyngeal wall and delayed reflex	Chin down	Pushes tongue base backward toward pharyngeal wall
Poor laryngeal protection	Chin down	Places extrinsic pressure on thyroid cartilage, increasing adduction
Poor laryngeal protection	Chin down head rotated to damaged side	Narrows laryngeal entrance and puts epiglottis in more protective position and increases vocal fold closure by applying extrinsic pressure
Delayed triggering of deglutition reflex	Tilt head forward	Prevents fluids from arriving at pharynx prematurely
Delayed triggering of swallow reflex	Effortful chin down	Forces the tongue backward to touch the faucial pillars
Impaired pharyngeal propulsive movements	Change of volume and viscosity	Thin liquids require less propulsive function force to move through pharynx
Difficulties in clearing oral cavity	Head back	Utilizes gravity
Residues in the pyriform sinus	Head rotated to damaged side	Helps unilateral laryngeal dysfunction
Food stuck	Head rotated to damaged side	Eliminates damaged side from bolus patch
Difficulties in manipulating the bolus on the weak side	Head tilt to stronger side	Directs bolus down stronger side
Impaired bolus formation	Strengthens weakened muscle	Controls lip and tongue movement
Impaired laryngeal closure	Supraglottic swallow	Helps laryngeal closure and swallow apnea
Impaired laryngeal closure	Strengthens weakened muscle	Laryngeal closure
Lying down on one side	Pharyngeal contraction and gravitational effects	Reduced pharyngeal contraction, eliminates gravitational effect, and helps to clean the residue on one side of pharynx
Poor oral or tongue control	Use of thickened liquids	Thickened liquids and pureed will not flow into larynx before it is protected
Poor tongue movement	Tilt head backward	Uses gravity to get bolus to pharynx
Unilateral pharyngeal/laryngeal paresis	Turn head to the affected side	Helps close larynx and/or pyriform sinus or the laryngeal sinus on the impaired/paretic (weak) side; bolus is directed along normal side

(indicated by a delay in onset of airway protection), a simple chin tuck reduces the speed of bolus passage, thereby giving the neural system the time it needs to initiate the pharyngeal and airway protection events prior to bolus entry.

Older individuals and especially those with dysphagia take longer to eat. Eating an adequate amount of food becomes a challenge not only because of the increased time required to do so but also because fatigue frequently becomes an issue. To promote a safe, efficient swallow in most individuals with swallowing and chewing difficulties, the following recommendations are useful:

- Alternate liquids and solids to "wash down" residue.
- Avoid mixing food and liquid in the same mouthful.
- Single textures are easier to eat.
- Concentrate on swallowing only.
- Eliminate distractions.
- Do not eat or drink when rushed or tired.
- Eat slowly to implement control of bolus flow and allow enough time for a meal.
- Place the food on the stronger side of the mouth if there is unilateral weakness.
- Avoid small food particles because they enter the airway more easily.
- Swallow than multiple textures.
- Take small amounts of food or liquid into the mouth.
- Use a teaspoon rather than a fork.
- Use sauces, condiments and gravies to facilitate cohesive bolus formation and to prevent aspiration.

Eating and drinking aids can assist in placing, directing, and controlling the bolus of food or liquid and in maintaining proper head posture while eating. For example, modified cups with cutout rims (placed over the bridge of the nose) or the use of straws prevent a backward head tilt when drinking to the bottom of a cup. A backward head tilt, which results in neck extension, should be avoided in most cases because food and liquid are more likely to be misdirected into the airway. Spoons with narrow, shallow bowls or glossectomy feeding spoons (spoons developed for moving food to the back of the tongue) are useful for individuals who require assistance in placing food in certain locations in the mouth. More importantly, these utensils and devices promote independence in eating and drinking. A speech pathologist can make suggestions about appropriate aids for optimizing swallowing safety and satisfaction. Occupational therapists are experts in the area of adaptive equipment and can help obtain products that are often available commercially. Diet modification is the most common compensatory intervention and is a totally passive environmental adaptation. Withholding thin liquids such as water, tea, or coffee, which are very easily aspirated by older adults, and restricting liquid intake to thickened liquids are almost routine in nursing homes in an attempt to minimize or eliminate thin liquid aspiration, presumably the precedent to the long-term-related outcome, i.e., pneumonia. Increasing the viscosity of liquids using thickener additives decreases the rate of flow and allows patients more time to initiate airway protection and prevents or decreases aspiration. Rehabilitative exercises are more active and rigorous than alternative interventions for dysphagia. Traditionally, a rehabilitative approach to dysphagia intervention has been withheld from older patients because such a demanding activity has been assumed to deplete any limited remaining swallowing reserve, thus potentially exacerbating dysphagia symptoms. The super-supraglottic swallow, effortful swallow, Mendelsohn maneuver, and the tongue-hold or Masako maneuver, as well as the Shaker exercise are examples of exercises requiring direct patient participation. Use of the supraglottic swallow increases airway protection as does a chin tuck position. Adaptive equipment (small-bowled spoon, shortened straw, cups with extended lip, and so forth) is used to control bolus size and allow midline introduction of bolus decreasing labial leakage. Modification of food consistencies and viscosity of liquids may also be recommended (e.g., puree, soft mechanical, thickened liquids). If it is determined that a patient is not a candidate for oral feeding, alternative means of nutritional support must be considered (nasogastric tube, percutaneous).

The *Shaker exercise*, which involves the patient lying flat and holding head and neck flexed forward while looking toward their feet, works to strengthen the muscles that open and close the esophageal sphincter, a muscle often weaker in older people.

Thermal-tactile stimulation involves use of a laryngeal mirror or probe dipped in ice and then presented to the faucial pillars to trigger pharyngeal constriction. This technique incorporates tactile and thermal modalities to affect a constriction and thus increase muscle strength and function. Other newer techniques, which may prove of additional therapeutic benefit following additional research and study, involve electrical stimulation of the swallowing musculature and pharyngeal muscle stimulation via lemon glycerin swabs. If treatment and compensatory strategies are not wholly effective, individuals may require thickened liquids to ensure safe swallowing; foods should also be chopped or ground to achieve optimal safety. Those with esophageal disorders may find thinner liquids more optimal for swallow function.

It has been determined that residue from above the glottis causes dysphagia and subsequent aspiration; the supraglottic swallow technique may be effective in clearing this residue. In this technique, the patient may be instructed to take a deep breath prior to swallowing. The patient then swallows, coughs, and swallows a second time before breathing again. If, on examination, pharyngeal weakness is evidenced unilaterally (most often this occurs following a stroke), the patient is instructed to turn his or her head to the weaker side thus compressing the area and helping prevent residue remaining on the weaker side. Similarly, tucking the chin can compress the valleculae and reduce residue risk in that area. Other individuals may require multiple swallows to achieve optimal swallow safety, due to generally weakened musculature [8].

Recent research on the benefits of lingual resistance exercise suggests that strength-building exercises for the tongue increase lingual muscle strength and mass and improve the timing of the swallowing components in healthy older adults, with implications for greater gains and carryover into swallowing-related outcomes in older dysphagic patients. The two exercise regimens described below, supported with efficacy data, improve swallowing function with the related outcome in older people. One is a simple isotonic/isometric neck exercise performed over a 6-week period in which the patient simply lies flat on his back and lifts his head (keeping shoulders flat) for a specified number of repetitions. The improved physiologic outcome of upper esophageal sphincter (UES) opening that affects swallowing is speculated to result from strengthening the mylohyoid/geniohyoid muscle groups and possibly the anterior segment of the digastric muscle. Another exercise program that is effective in older dysphagic patients comprises an 8-week isometric resistance exercise for the tongue and related oropharyngeal musculature.

In summary, while oropharyngeal dysphagia may be life threatening, so are some of the alternatives, particularly for frail older patients. Therefore, contributions by all team members are valuable in this challenging decision-making process, in which the opinion of the patient's family or care provider is perhaps the most critical. The evidence calls for more research, including randomized clinical trials in this area. Until (and perhaps after) these data are collected and have been analyzed, the many behavioral, dietary, and environmental modifications described in this manuscript are compassionate and, in many cases, preferred alternatives to the always present option of tube feeding.

In terms of older people with dementia in assisted living or old-age homes, a number of studies indicating that indirect interventions, e.g., improving the environment, exploiting food preferences, reducing distractions, touch and caregiver interaction, all facilitate increased nutritional intake. Hotaling [24] discusses the important influences that the environment has on preparing residents for eating and describes some of the environmental factors that promote a positive mealtime experience for residents. Tube feeding is also used where nutritional intake is poor because of cognitive impairment. The initiation of tube feeding, particularly in the latter group, is often fraught with ethical and moral dilemmas, and much debate as to the indications and contraindications of tube feeding in these groups has been addressed in the literature [25]. Behavioral modifications, postural adjustments, and training of caregivers in feeding techniques are equally important in the management of the dysphagic patient. In our study, the doctor's recommendations on feeding modality in patients diagnosed to have unsafe swallows were based on the assumption that the degree of swallowing dysfunction (and the corresponding risk of aspiration) was reflected in the number of abnormal findings found in bedside assessment. In comparison, the speech therapist's recommendations also took into consideration other factors such as the phase of swallowing affected in dysphagia, the patient's ability to comprehend instructions, and the patient's ability to participate in behavioral and postural modifications.

Clinical Cases

Case A

We report a clinical case of an 81-year-old lady (Mrs. A.), admitted to a long-term care (LTC) facility for rehabilitation due to a hospital immobilization syndrome developed as a complication of fractures involving multiple regions of one lower limb. The patient's clinical history included a depressive status (Geriatric Depression Scale 8/15), difficulties to respond to orders, and moderate memory impairment probably due to sensorial deprivation and lack of stimulation during hospitalization. The Mini Mental Examination showed a moderate cognitive impairment (22/30), and the nutritional assessment indicated risk of dehydration and malnutrition. Initially, the patient scored a Barthel of 60/100, which indicates moderate dependency for the activities of daily living. She still had the ability to eat and drink all the consistencies through the mouth independently, despite taking a long time to eat.

When Mrs. A. was admitted to the LTC facility, she was clinically stable with no acute symptoms of the brain or other acute organ disease. No anterior history of stroke or other neurological diseases that can cause dysphagia were reported except a progressive, non-asymptomatic encephalopathy. However, the decline of functional status and the state of dependency were clear, thus making her eligible for an appropriate individual plan of rehabilitation including for swallowing and nutrition. Due to medication, she also showed xerostomy that compromised the preparatory and the oral phase of swallow.

The patient was assessed for dysphagia with the Mann Assessment Swallowing Ability (MASA) and also performed the 3-oz water swallow test. A moderate problem in the preparatory phase of swallowing was identified demonstrating food retention inside the mouth. When performing the 3-oz water swallow test, she coughed and showed wet voice two seconds after the water swallow was completed.

Suddenly, five days after LTC admission, the patient began to cough during lunch, describing it as food stuck and difficulty in respiratory control. Mrs. A also showed difficulty in retaining food inside the mouth, swallow stages coordination, and bolus propulsion from the mouth into the pharynx. No respiratory complications were observed in the subsequent days, but signs of laryngeal penetration were each day more frequent.

After this episode, the patient's oral assessment and examination showed poor control of the tongue, tremor, lack of sensibility in the tongue and soft palate, with an impairment of coordination of global oral movements.

Regarding the patient's complaints, she mentioned a progressive decline, throughout the hospitalization, of oral mobility including tongue strength with poor nutrition intake although no important weight loss was referred. Furthermore, many attempts to trigger the swallow reflex were observed, even with saliva. All these problems together made it more difficult for her to manage the bolus preparation and propulsion, especially with food with different consistencies. The flexible endoscopic examination confirmed a swallowing disturbance with food and liquid stagnation in the glossoepiglottic valleculae and penetrations of food and liquids with a cough reflex mechanism moderately effective.

Due the aforementioned progressive encephalopathy, Mrs. A was diagnosed with neurogenic dysphagia that compromises all the swallow stages including sensory tongue receptors.

Since the patient showed a moderate comorbidity and disability status and a moderate dysphagia (initially undiagnosed), a speech therapy and rehabilitation program were considered appropriate in order to enhance organ effectiveness and regain efficiency in all the swallowing function. An appropriate nutritional program with adequate dietary recommendations and changes (avoiding mixed consistencies and stimulating the taste) was applied. Compensatory strategies (such as body and neck posture changes) were taught to the patient in order to improve her swallowing performance and regain confidence.

In this case, the immobilization syndrome was an aggravating factor cumulated to the predisposing neurogenic dysphagia due to the progressive encephalopathy. Moreover, the mild cognitive impairment, sensory deprivation, and frailty, which result in low awareness of the problem by the patient with maladaptive and excessive fear of gagging, results in poor food intake enhancing the state of weakness and the risk of laryngeal penetration and aspiration.

Case B

Mr. S. was an 80-year-old male living alone in his own house receiving formal day care for medication and for some instrumental activities of daily living including meal preparation. The patient's clinical exam by the physician described a high consumption of alcohol for many years with no history of previous stroke or other neurogenic progressive disorders. Signs of generalized encephalopathy were detected in a CT scan. The Barthel Index scored 80/100, which indicates mild dependency. He still maintained the ability to eat alone. However, the oral intake was poor. A status of sarcopenia was assessed with handgrip performance below the normal age and sex-matched references. A secondary sarcopenia was diagnosed, which results from inactivity, comorbid conditions, and malnutrition. Mr. S. used to stay in bed during a large part of the day, showing difficulties in basic movements such as walking short distances and remaining seated in a chair. Due to inactivity, age-related conditions, and comorbidities, Mr. S. showed loss of muscle mass and function and was accompanied by weight loss. He became apathetic, experienced decline in cognitive capacity and global motor skills, and began to demonstrate difficulty in the maintenance of adequate social relationships. The clinical profile for Mr. S. indicates global physical, cognitive, and social deterioration.

The swallowing assessment showed vallecular and pyriform sinus residues after swallowing and changes in the activity patterns in the tongue, soft palate, and suprahyoid muscles. Mr. S. also showed changes in swallow respiratory coordination, due to decreased muscle mobility and/or reaction times compromising swallowing apnea and airway protection. In this case, age-related changes of swallowing function potentiated by the secondary sarcopenia amplified the penetration/aspiration risk due to diminished functional reserve of the head, neck, and respiratory muscles. This situation cumulated with the comorbidity status due to life-long alcohol abuse and polymedication.

Nutrition was compromised by the difficulties of limited mobility and even difficulty in opening the recipients that contained the meals and transport food into the mouth. Physical constraints add to poor appetite, weight loss, and dehydration. The patient also mentioned changes in smell and taste probably due to the decline in the density of tongue sensory organs which resulted in taste dysfunction and the decline in the pleasure to appreciate food.

Mr. S. was thus eligible for an appropriate individual day care plan of rehabilitation, including swallowing and nutrition, as well as adaptive techniques that included adequate dietary intake, following the basic principle of dysphagia rehabilitation. The physical therapist and the speech and language therapist work together in a daily basis in order to implement a program of strength-training exercises. After 8 weeks, Mr. S improved general force capacity, increased functional reserve which allowed him to participate in extended task-specific exercises including oral motor organs, implemented as a complementary therapy to task-specific swallowing practice. A tongue and facial organ resistance program (motor exercises to increase muscle strength and range of motion in oropharyngeal structures) was enacted simultaneously with global motor exercises of the upper and lower limbs, balance, and endurance. Sensory-based swallowing therapies that aim to increase taste and motor response were performed.

Mr. S. showed a significant increase in all the swallowing process after three months of speech therapy with a better lingual propulsion, more efficient suprahyoid muscle movements, better laryngeal protection, and diminishing the residues. Compensatory strategies were used to alter the propulsion of material into the pharynx especially for liquids. Chin down and head rotation decreased significantly laryngeal penetration which results in more confidence when swallowing.

Consent

The patients gave written informed consent to describe their clinical cases.

Bibliography

1. Eurostat. Population projections 2004–2050. Eurostat; 2005. p. 6. Eurostat Press Office, Luxembourg http://europa.eu.int/comm/eurostat/
2. Ginocchio D, Borghi C, Schindler A. Dysphagia assessment in the elderly. Nutr Ther Metab. 2009;27(1):9–15.
3. Roy N, Stemple J, Merrill RM, Thomas L. Dysphagia in the elderly: preliminary evidence of prevalence, risk factors, and socioemotional effects. Ann Otol Rhinol Laryngol. 2007;116(11): 858–65.
4. Chouinard J, Lavigne E, Villeneuve C. Weight loss, dysphagia, and outcome in advanced dementia. Dysphagia. 1998;13(3):151–5.
5. Schindler O, Ruoppolo G, Schindler A. Deglutologia. Milano: Omega Edizione; 2011.
6. Schindler JS, Kelly JH. Swallowing disorders in the elderly. Laryngoscope. 2002;112(4): 589–602.
7. Paterson WG. Dysphagia in the elderly. Can Fam Physician. 1996;42:925–32.
8. Prasse J, Kikano J. An overview of dysphagia in the elderly. Adv Stud Med. 2004;4(10): 527–33.
9. Yoshikawa M, Yoshida M, Nagasaki T, Tanimoto K, Tsuga K, Akagawa Y. Effects of tooth loss and denture wear on tongue-tip motion in elderly dentulous and edentulous people. J Oral Rehabil. 2008;35(12):882–8.
10. Youmans SR, Youmans GL, Stierwalt JA. Differences in tongue strength across age and gender: is there a diminished strength reserve? Dysphagia. 2009;24(1):57–65.

11. Kikutani T, Tamura F, Nishiwaki K, Kodama M, Suda M, Fukui T, et al. Oral motor function and masticatory performance in the community-dwelling elderly. Odontology. 2009;97(1):38–42.

12. Logemann JA, Pauloski BR, Rademaker AW, Colangelo LA, Kahrilas PJ, Smith CH. Temporal and biomechanical characteristics of oropharyngeal swallow in younger and older men. J Speech Lang Hear Res. 2000;43(5):1264–74.

13. Doty RW, Bosma JF. An electromyographic analysis of reflex deglutition. J Neurophysiol. 1956;19(1):44–60.

14. Allepaerts S, Delcourt S, Petermans J. Swallowing disorders in the elderly: an underestimated problem. Rev Med Liege. 2008;63(12):715–21.

15. Miura H, Kariyasu M, Yamasaki K, Arai Y. Evaluation of chewing and swallowing disorders among frail community-dwelling elderly individuals. J Oral Rehabil. 2007;34(6):422–7.

16. Ashley J, Duggan M, Sutcliffe N. Speech, language, and swallowing disorders in the older adult. Clin Geriatr Med. 2006;22(2):291–310, viii.

17. Burda AN. Communication and swallowing changes in healthy aging adults. Iowa: Jones&bartlett Leraning; 2011.

18. Schindler A, Ginocchio D, Ruoppolo G. What we don't know about dysphagia complications? Rev Laryngol Otol Rhinol (Bord). 2008;129(2):75–8.

19. Oguchi K, Saitoh E, Baba M, Kusudo S. The Repetitive Saliva Swallowing Test (RSST) as a Screening Test of Functional Dysphagia Validity of RSST. Jpn J Rehabil Med. 2000;37(6):383–8.

20. DePippo KL, Holas MA, Reding MJ. Validation of the 3-oz water swallow test for aspiration following stroke. Arch Neurol. 1992;49(12):1259–61.

21. Wilkins T, Gillies RA, Thomas AM, Wagner PJ. The prevalence of dysphagia in primary care patients: a HamesNet Research Network study. J Am Board Family Med. 2007;20(2):144–50.

22. O'Loughlin G, Shanley C. Swallowing problems in the nursing home: a novel training response. Dysphagia. 1998;13(3):172–83.

23. Mepani R, Antonik S, Massey B, Kern M, Logemann J, Pauloski B, et al. Augmentation of deglutitive thyrohyoid muscle shortening by the Shaker Exercise. Dysphagia. 2009;24(1):26–31.

24. Hotaling DL. Nutritional considerations for the pureed diet texture in dysphagic elderly. Dysphagia. 1992;7(2):81–5.

25. Chen PH, Golub JS, Hapner ER, Johns 3rd MM. Prevalence of perceived dysphagia and quality-of-life impairment in a geriatric population. Dysphagia. 2009;24(1):1–6.

Printed in the United States
By Bookmasters